MW01294914

Autism:

44 Ways to Understanding - Aspergers Syndrome, ADHD, ADHD, and Special Needs

Margaret LaRue

Copyright 2015 by Margaret LaRue - All rights reserved.

This document is geared towards providing exact and reliable information in regards to the topic and issue covered. The publication is sold with the idea that the publisher is not required to render accounting, officially permitted, or otherwise, qualified services. If advice is necessary, legal or professional, a practiced individual in the profession should be ordered.

- From a Declaration of Principles which was accepted and approved equally by a Committee of the American Bar Association and a Committee of Publishers and Associations.

In no way is it legal to reproduce, duplicate, or transmit any part of this document in either electronic means or in printed format. Recording of this publication is strictly prohibited and any storage of this document is not allowed unless with written permission from the publisher. All rights reserved.

The information provided herein is stated to be truthful and consistent, in that any liability, in terms of inattention or otherwise, by any usage or abuse of any policies, processes, or directions contained within is the solitary and utter responsibility of the recipient reader. Under no circumstances will any legal responsibility or blame be held against the publisher for any reparation, damages, or monetary loss due to the information herein, either directly or indirectly.

Respective authors own all copyrights not held by the publisher.

The information herein is offered for informational purposes solely, and is universal as so. The presentation of the information is without contract or any type of guarantee assurance.

The trademarks that are used are without any consent, and the publication of the trademark is without permission or backing by the trademark owner. All trademarks and brands within this book are for clarifying purposes only and are the owned by the owners themselves, not affiliated with this document.

TABLE OF CONTENTS

INTRODUCTION

I want to thank you for reading this book, *Autism: 44 Ways to Understanding- Asperger's Syndrome, ADHD, ADHD, and Special Needs.*

Life with special needs children and adults can be both challenging and deeply rewarding. For many, though, there's a learning curve involved that's relatively steep, so I've written this book in the hope of offering some concrete help to those of you struggling to make sense of life with the special needs and differently calibrated people in your life.

It may be that you're reading this book as a way of better understanding yourself as a special needs person. In that case, I hope you find some encouragement here and some ways and means of better managing your symptoms.

This book contains proven steps and strategies about how to help you cope with, understand, and communicate with people who have "unique learning abilities". These include people with Asperger's (also known as Asperger's Syndrome), Attention-Deficit/Hyperactivity Disorder (ADHD), and autism. Both children and adults live with the challenges of these conditions. There are actually more than 44 ways to achieve this in this book, but I thought 44 had a nice ring to it. I'd like this book to give you the tools you need to help you understand, cope, live with, and enjoy the ones close to you, dealing with any of these conditions.

This book is intended to provide you a solid foundation from which you can build a greater understanding of either yourself, or your loved ones with these and other conditions. I hope it helps you relate to those who need to be understood the most. The strategies detailed in this book will help to arm you with the best ways to care for, educate, communicate, and better love those who depend on you. Like everyone else, children and adults with special needs seek to be understood. By following the advice I've outlined, I hope you'll be able to offer the gift of loving understanding to your special needs love one.

Thanks again for reading this book, I hope you enjoy it!

CHAPTER 1

ASPERGER'S SYNDROME: DEFINITION AND SYMPTOMS

What is Asperger's Syndrome?

Asperger Syndrome is an autism spectrum disorder (ASD) affecting both children and adults. People with Asperger's Syndrome find it challenging to interact with other people, especially in social settings. Often they do not understand the meaning behind different emotions, and therefore can't react properly (or in what is considered to be a "socially acceptable" manner) to situations implicating the emotions of others.

For example, a teenager with Asperger Syndrome may not understand the need to engage in small talk with his classmates, especially in between lessons. Or the other extreme may be the case. A person with AS may be too self-focused and unconcerned about the opinion of others, and so, talk incessantly about personal interests and obsessions. Either way, this teen would end up being isolated from his peer group, leading to greater confusion and social awkwardness. These habits can be carried into adulthood and cause significant problems in professional life, as well as romantic relationships friendships and family life.

Aspergers' Syndrome does not cause significant difficulties in a person's cognitive development. This means that a person suffering from it is rarely prone to stuttering or delayed understanding of the world. In fact, many people with Asperger's Syndrome exhibit high intelligence or specialty in a specific field. Data science, IT and analytical professionals like polling tend to be good matches for adults with AS, because they utilize the particularity of AS focus. Asperger's adults are also at home in engineering, computer sciences, and as librarians and accounting. Their attention to detail is legendary and any of these professional areas are highly suited to this aspect of Asperger's.

Symptoms of Asperger's Syndrome

Below are the common symptoms of Asperger's Syndrome. Please note that not all of these are always present in the same person, making it difficult to diagnose the condition at an early age:

1. Discomfort in social settings and the inability to communicate adequately or appropriately with other people. AS children tend not to be able to express themselves in a manner found coherent by most people. Because of this factor, they often find it difficult to say what's on their minds or express in a way that other people consider normative, or are able to comprehend. Whether children or adults, AS sufferers generally encounter a high level of social anxiety, which may cause them to act out in social settings.

2. AS people are often interpreted by others to be self-centered and uncaring about other people's opinions and situations. This means they misinterpret other people's needs and appear to be lost in their own world. While it's not their intention, AS people tend not to understand the concept of dialogue, preferring one-way conversations about their personal interests and obsessions. This is due to the focus AS people enjoy. Asperger's allows those who live with it to become highly knowledgeable about pet subjects. They're only too happy to recite their knowledge as though lecturing, completely unaware that others are disengaging. AS people have difficulty making space for others to speak, especially when they're on a roll.

This is not a lack of concern. This is just a facet of AS.

3. AS people also have an inability to "read between the lines," especially in terms of body language and non-verbal cues. This is one of the most prominent symptoms with Asperger's syndrome. AS people will not understand things unless they're specifically and clearly explained to them. They are not capable of understanding nuance and will not be able to decipher clues. They need a clear exposition of what's under discussion, with no grey areas and tend not to understand when humor is in play, sarcasm, or innuendo.

4. AS people have a tendency to be tactless and frank to the point of being rude. This is because they don't have the capacity to hold back opinions and will be straightforward about anything and everything being discussed. They have no filters. Once you get accustomed to this aspect of AS, it will seem less odd, but many people have difficulty interacting with AS people because of it. They blurt things out, make comments that aren't considered appropriate, may laugh inappropriately and generally seem to others like the proverbial bull in a china shop.

5. A common feature of AS is difficulty making eye contact, or having conversations face to face. AS people tend to be shy and more importantly, lack the confidence to engage in what are widely considered to be normal conversations with people. They know they're different. They're just not sure why. They prefer to answer with a simple "yes" or "no", without elaborating on their response. This is especially true if they are not interested in speaking with the person that is trying to hold the conversation with them. This isn't contempt or rudeness. It's just a simple fact. If what you're saying bores the AS person you're talking to, they will tune out and think about their personal interests while you're speaking.

6. Repetitive speech patterns are common to people with Asperger's. They tend to repeat the same statements until they are satisfied and won't stop doing so, even if they are asked to stop. This is their way of working through a problem (thinking out loud is also quite common), or formulating a more complete thought from an idea they've had.

7. AS people very commonly have difficulty in maintaining relationships. They often have recurring problems that can deter them from maintaining health friendships, romantic and professional relationships. The mood swings and emotional outbursts some Asperger's people are prone to can make life very difficult for life partners, family, friends and co-workers. Some people throw their hands up in despair and simply walk away.

8. Their excellence in verbal skills can often mask the commonly poor nonverbal communication skills most AS people struggle with. They are able to converse extremely well and usually have large vocabularies, but their difficulty with reading body language, nuance and non-verbal cues. Nodding, shaking hands and waving are all foreign to AS people, who tend not to like physical contact, particularly in public setting, and prefer to begin the conversation immediately, even while approaching the person they intend to converse with, from a distance.

Diagnosing Asperger's Syndrome

Asperger Syndrome is a bit trickier to diagnose in comparison to to other ASDs. This is especially true of teenagers, who may appear to be undergoing one of the phases adolescents are so prone to.

The key to assisting a person suffering from Asperger Syndrome is to diagnose the condition as early as possible and to come up with a program or treatment for that person. But in order to do so, one must keep an eye out for the symptoms and determine whether they are caused by Asperger's or by another disorder, such as ADHD. The symptoms of these two conditions are very similar. Indeed, some medical professionals make the mistake of diagnosing AS people with a different type of autism, only to find out later that the patient, in fact, has Asperger's. This can result in inappropriate medication being prescribed, which can lead to some disastrous results, including exacerbating existing symptoms.

If you believe a loved one or friend has Asperger's Syndrome, you should carefully watch for signs or symptoms to confirm that you're not leading this person to a misdiagnosis. Remember that the perceptions of loved ones can weigh heavily in arriving at a diagnosis. Be as clear about what you're seeing as possible and perhaps, keep a symptom journal to show the clinical practitioner who will make the diagnosis. Watch your loved one's social interactions closely. You can do this without being obvious about it. Look for signs that your friend or family member is struggling with autism, paying special attention to whether they're displaying any of the symptoms listed above.

Since people with Asperger's Syndrome often have a specialty or a unique skill, it's also advisable to look out for talents or obsessions that may contribute to the social awkwardness of a potential patient, due to the perceptions of others with regard to this habit. Obsessive focus on any one subject or area of interest can indicate Asperger's, particularly when that subject or interest is the topic of every conversation the AS person engages on. When this occurs regularly, causing others to avoid interacting with the person involved, you may want to consult a clinician toward seeking a diagnosis. It's one of the most compelling hallmarks of the condition.

CHAPTER 2

TIPS ON DEALING WITH PEOPLE WITH ASPERGER'S SYNDROME

I have spent considerable time in the company of a person with Asperger's Syndrome. This was not in a clinical or professional setting. Rather, I was married to an undiagnosed person with AS.

Life with Kendall

High strung, fast-talking, highly intelligent and oddly focused on topics that would sometimes drive those around him to distraction, Kendall is one of the most intelligent people I have ever known. I fell irretrievably in love with him, over time. He was different from other men I'd known and had an old-fashioned, almost courtly air about. For instance, he would never hold my hand in public. He would ask that I rest my hand in the crook of his arm. I found this both quaintly old timey and adorable.

Kendall and I took our time on the road to marriage and enjoyed a long engagement. During this time, we co-habited. We sought out a home that suited us both and proceeded toward the altar with no little caution. I wanted to be absolutely sure I was making the right decision and that meant understanding Kendall in a domestic setting. People have been known to change once living under the same roof and Kendall was no exception.

While we'd been dating, I'd often been frustrated by his refusal to permit to visit his apartment. He always made me wait in the car when he stopped by to fetch something. Finally, I coaxed him into letting me come in with him. All the way to the door, he apologized for the state he'd left it in. I reassured him it was fine with me; that I didn't care.

But when Kendall opened the door to his apartment, the sight that greeted me was nothing short of appalling. Clothes lay in heaps everywhere. Dishes were piled in the sink. Uneaten food littered the countertops. I won't even describe the bed. It was just more of the same. The effect was that of a hoarder with nothing to hoard except a pervasive disorder that extended from one end of the place to the other. Kendall's apartment looked like a fourteen-year-old's bedroom.

Small wonder he'd been reluctant to permit me to enter.

I should have known nothing would change as far as his personal habits were concerned, once we moved in together. Nothing did change. If anything, he became more resolutely neglectful, throwing his clothes on the floor of our shared office when returning home from his job as an IT specialist. Each night, he would wander distractedly into the living room, wearing the same crusty pair of track pants. When I'd attempt to wash these, he would object, insisting they weren't that dirty. They were.

But I had no idea what the problem with was Kendall. I was unfamiliar with the ASD spectrum at the time, so I chalked his behavior up to personality quirks and a nervous disposition. In short – I loved him, so I worked around it.

I managed to prevent entropy from setting it for the first two years of our lives together, diligently maintaining our home in as orderly a state as I possibly could, under the circumstances. My free time was devoted to rounding up stray dishes, cups and glasses, abandoned in every room of the house, including the washroom dedicated to his use (for it was not possible for anyone on earth to share a washroom with Kendall, due to the horrific disarray in which he maintained it).

Had I not pursued the maintenance of our mutual home, things would have been much worse. Eventually, though, other life priorities took over. My studies and other activities precluded my vain attempts at preventing the encroachment of total chaos and so were limited to a frenzied effort, once per week. In the meantime, my entreaties for him to help were ignored.

Lost articles of clothing, lost keys, lost wallets, lost cellular phones (you name it) were frequent interruptions in the course of our daily lives. Losing one of these items would provoke a meltdown, involving throwing items from shelves in order to find it. I would stand by helplessly, as Kendall proceeded to tear the house apart, yelling at the top of his lungs. Sometimes the frustration would be too much for him and a piece of furniture would be broken. At times, these tantrums were frightening to watch, but there was nothing I could do to stop them. Once Kendall had spiraled into one of his outbursts, all I could do was wait for it to end.

Following our wedding, things became increasingly worse, as I struggled to help him control his outbursts and maintain his things in some kind of order. From time to time, his mother would come by to help with organizing his clothes. At one point, I approached her to see what might be done about Kendall's behavior, but she insisted it was his personality and that nothing could be done about it. She had no interest in facing whatever was at the root of his behavior.

The tantrums continued and were no longer private, but sometimes thrown in professional or social settings. My friends stopped coming around, or calling. They couldn't cope with the lengthy monologues he engaged in, or his continual interruptions when they attempted to change the subject to something that might interest everyone present.

Over the years of our marriage, a string of lost jobs, ruined vacations and strained friendships marked our lives together. On several occasions, I left to stay at a friend's home, when the pressure had built to the breaking point. I found myself finding excuses to be out of the house, doing other things. I could no longer cope with Kendall's behavior, which bordered on spousal abuse.

Finally, I arranged to take him to see a counsellor (with the intervention of a mutual friend). In only one session, his condition was identified as Asperger's. The relief was immediate. For years, Kendall had suffered from his symptoms in varying degrees, beginning in childhood. Having observed his father, it seemed they were both afflicted, although Kendall's father had never been diagnosed. For awhile, life became easier.

But then, another job loss came. This had involved a workplace meltdown. Then other stressors, piled one upon the other. Money worries, car troubles, family issues. The dam finally burst and I called a friend to help me move my things from our home.

Several weeks later, Kendall agreed to try medication. His behavior and symptoms were so greatly improved by this therapy I agreed to move back in. All was well, until the medication ran out and Kendall refused to renew the prescription. Try as I might, he resisted. His defiance and belligerence in the matter led to the worst of all the blow ups I'd ever seen him have. I asked him to leave the house and after several days, demanded a divorce.

My life with Kendall will sound familiar to others who have been married to people with Asperger's. The chaos could flare up at any moment. The instability of our lives was under constant threat of a meltdown or outburst. This prevented me from feeling at ease in his presence. It was as though I was always walking on eggshells, trying to keep the peace. If you've been there, you'll recognize everything I'm talking about.

To this day, I regret not having been better equipped to deal with Kendall and his symptoms. I did what I could, though and I hope he has finally pursued treatment, for his own sake. My life with Kendall is another motivation for writing this book. I want to help others prevent at least some of what I went through, due to the fact I had no idea what I was dealing with.

How You Can Help

Someone with Asperger's Syndrome needs all the love and support you and the immediate circle of family and friends can provide. Part of that is accepting the fact there might be a problem. In my case, Kendall's family had no interest in discussing the possibility there might be a clinical reason underlying his behavior. They simply wouldn't hear it.

Support and patience are even more urgently needed for children and teenagers with the condition, as people in these age groups are already coping with the project of growing up. While these epochs of our lives can be joyful, they can also be painful and confusing. Just add AS to make it that much more so. Older patients may deal the condition more effectively, but may also suffer from factors unique to adulthood, like difficulty with romantic and professional relationships. Kendall's difficulties had begun in childhood and, never having been addressed, continued into adulthood, where they caused him to lose jobs, friendships and ultimately his marriage.

If you have a loved one with Asperger's, it is essential that you provide emotional support and a great deal of patience. I did what I could in my situation, but without any knowledge of the condition, I was not equipped to support Kendall effectively. Even following diagnosis, the lack of support from family and friends (as they didn't know any more about AS than I did) exacerbated the situation.

Remember that most of your AS loved one's actions are based on a lack of understanding about how social norms and their unwritten rules, and how they apply. It's not just stubbornness or pigheadedness. The AS person is genuinely lost when it comes to the ins and outs of social engagement and needs to be lead through that wilderness with an understanding hand.

Following are twenty tips you can follow to help you deal with a loved one with Asperger's Syndrome:

1. **Have a regular schedule.** Routine is an important part of life for a person with Asperger's Syndrome. Having specific tasks to perform at set times of the day can help AS people maintain much-needed equilibrium. Routine is beloved by those with AS and providing a framework that encourages routine is a great life support. Try to set a standard time for everyday activities—meals, homework, leisure—and stick to it. If you are dealing with a child or teenager with Asperger's, you can set a regular bedtime and list of daily chores, too. You have to stress the importance of a timetable, every day, in order for your AS loved one to feel comfortable and at home in the family's environment and also, an integral part of it. With time, your AS loved one will become accustomed to performing certain tasks at designated times. This will be a welcome source of the routine and structure so highly prized by people with this condition. Without family and clinical support, though, it will be very difficult to obtain your AS loved one's cooperation, if they're an adult. AS people can be extraordinarily stubborn, believing that they're always the smartest person in the room. They need a very good, rational reason to modify their behavior and it's often the case that one person telling them they need to modify their behavior is not going to cut it.

2. **Be patient.** A person with Asperger's Syndrome, especially if a child, is rarely aware others can be impacted by words and actions common to the condition. Your patience, tolerance and understanding of the tactlessness, temper tantrums, and mood swings common to AS are strongly advised. Kindness and compassion for your loved one's condition should be

accompanied by the management of your own expectations. Being ever mindful of the fact that AS people see and live in the world in a very unique way is the best place start, but this is something to be remembered at the start of each day. Impatience, shouting and attempting to discipline AS children and youth as you would other children, can leave a lasting and deleterious psychological impact. These young people are not the same and require special care. You might have to deal with bigger problems if you lose your temper with as AS youth, as AS people are known for acting out when frustrated, which can prompt impulsive or even violent behavior. As described above, Kendall was prone to breaking things when in the throes of a tantrum. While he was never physically abusive, the walls over our home had more than one scar and even one hole. He also punched a hole in the wall of a hospital at one point, due to his frustration over the condition of a family member.

Remember, children emulate the adults in their lives. They repeat the behaviors they see around them. Remaining as calm and unruffled as possible is the key to being your AS youth's best friend.

3. **Discipline and rebuke with love.** Discipline a child or teenager with Asperger's Syndrome if you must—but explain clearly why you are doing it, and remind your AS youth that discipline doesn't mean you don't love them. Quite the opposite. If you are dealing with an adult with the condition, don't hesitate to point out bad or rude behavior, but do so in a loving manner. Be clear about pointing out what the AS person did wrong, clearly and simply. Be prepared for a debate, as the AS person defends his behavior and enjoys the odd conflict in order to flex his verbal skills. In fact, this is something Kendall lived for. He never missed the opportunity to engage in an argument (with anyone available), often employing circuitous and repetitive arguments in order to wear the other party to the debate down.

Don't give in, though. Be firm. Add suggestions for how the behavior you're pointing out as wrong might be mitigated next time. This is helpful. Logic is always welcome by AS people, as it provides a clear roadmap from point A to point B. If even they resist, stick your guns. Eventually, you'll be able to budge them a little closer to where you want them to be. It may even be helpful to walk away from the conflict in order to give your AS loved one an opportunity to cool down and think about your side of the discussion.

4. **Build a reliable support group.** Nobody should have to take this journey alone. Living with a person with Asperger's Syndrome can drain you of your energy if you try to do it all by yourself. Get help—whether in the form of moral, emotional, or physical support (financial, even). Family members, friends, and colleagues that you trust can all be part of your network of support. I was very unfortunate in this regard. Kendall's family was unwilling to consider that he might have a clinical condition. His friends had grown accustomed to him to the point they couldn't understand why I was having difficulty coping with him. My friends commiserated, but were no more equipped than I was to cope. I had at least one friend, though, that was able to conspire with me to get him to a doctor and obtain a diagnosis and for this, I'd truly grateful.

Let the people in your support group be your sounding board for the difficulties you experience while learning to live with your loved one's condition and all it implies and brings with it. Allow them to help you with little things to lighten your load. If you don't have the makings of such a support network around you, you can reach out for counseling or therapy, which is what I did. This will help ease the daily stress of living with the condition. Also, a diagnosis is a tremendous relief to many people with AS, especially Aspies. Having spent their lives with the knowledge that something's not quite as it should be, knowing there's a name for it is somewhat comforting. It also provides a clearer idea of what might be done to mitigate the conditions effects. Remember that to help your loved learn to live more effectively with Asperger's, *your* mental and emotional state should also be stable and reliable. That was certainly not the case with me. I was so frazzled from dealing with years of Kendall's behavior and symptoms that I had lost the will to fight. I was burned out, exhausted and eventually, the lack of support from my network and Kendall's reluctance to undergo any kind of ongoing treatment broke this camel's back.

Your Asperger's loved on depends on your support. If you get sick, or burn out, you can't provide that. Some choose to suffer in silence, virtual martyrs to AS. But there is absolutely no need for that. You can open up to others to ease some of the pressure you may feel from time to time. You will be in a better position to help your AS loved one and work with their issues. So don't hold anything back and be honest about your daily struggles with Asperger's Syndrome with those around you, as this will better enable you to be the best possible partner to your AS loved one you possibly can. Support is absolutely crucial. If you don't get that, the consequences are clear enough from my example. I had no choice but to leave, as Kendall would not pursue any treatment or action to mitigate his symptoms. Frankly, at that point, it was either him or me and I chose me.

5. **Pick your battles.** Do not be quick to reprimand a person with Asperger's Syndrome, especially in the midst of an emotional outburst or episode of acting out. Opt to discuss your concerns openly, providing your AS loved one with options to choose from. This involves both parties in the discussion about what's to be done and empowers the AS person in your life to consider and take decisions rationally and deliberately. This practice builds much needed confidence. Lashing out instead of calmly discussing the matter is a much less successful path to resolving conflict with AS people and will probably make the situation worse. Generally speaking, your AS loved one will not even understand why you're upset, because Asperger's people don't

understand the emotional responses of others unless they're adequately explained. Don't let your emotions get the better of you. That's for you AS loved one! Sometimes, it best to let them melt right down to the quick, without intervening. They need to burn as hot as they're going to so you can have a rational, intelligent discussion with them. The heat of the moment is not the time for that.

6. **Prepare a ready set of verbal and physical cues.** Establish a set of codes that you and your loved one can use to help you quickly determine if either one of you needs something from the other. This also works if you feel that you are about to get angry, or that your loved one is about to throw a tantrum. Using verbal cues or gestures can help you take some time out from the conflict and defer discussion until both of you are in a better mood to talk about it. Holding up one hand (palm forward) in front of the other person's face is a good way to stop the conflict immediately. Both parties have to agree to this cue. Alternatively, a "safe word" can be used. You can choose a word that doesn't generally come up in the course of every day conversation. Let your AS love one choose this. Asperger's people have a love of language that will make this a fun project (although it may take some time, as the possibilities will have to be analyzed, categorized, sanforized and then discussed). A word like "glabrous", for example, might be the ideal choice and even defuse the conflict due to the sheer improbability and silliness of it cropping up in the middle of an argument. The word I frequently used with Kendall was "spiraling". When I sensed he was going into the dreaded spiral, I would say it very quietly, adding volume to the word, as the spiral continued. This would usually work if I caught the brewing tantrum before it had worked up a head of steam. Once the tipping point has come with an AS outburst, all the safe words and hand signals in the world aren't going to help. You have

to catch it as soon as the wind picks up, not when the tornado is already sucking cars into its vortex. Whatever you choose as your signal or word, make sure you're both fully on board. No bending the rules on this one. Your AS loved one may even like to formulate a brief form of contract to seal the deal. This might be another confidence-building and engrossing project to engage in and learn from.

7. **Be aware of stressors in the environment.** Take time to learn what may cause panic attacks, and prepare for them. These could be problems in school or at the office, peer pressure, or even a romantic issue. Have suggestions about emotional management on hand to help your AS loved one deal with them, and provide advice on how the stressor in play might best be dealt with. Prepare a list of the various external stressors and possible triggers you can identify in your loved one's various environments and keep tabs on how these are playing out, from time to time. Your loved one may not be able to express the emotional problem adequately and you may have to ask questions in order to know exactly what's happening and how you can help overcome the problem. A frequent trigger for Kendall involved driving and suddenly realizing he didn't know where he was because he'd been daydreaming, or because another driver had done something he disagreed with. This could lead to accidents, road rage and rolling arguments which might have been avoided with more awareness on my part. Learning about them, following diagnosis was a process and I became better at identifying his driving triggers as time when by.

8. **Don't beat up yourself up.** Everyone messes up sometimes. Nobody's perfect. This is a rule of life to keep at the forefront as you journey with your AS loved one. But don't blame yourself for the sudden panic attacks or because you occasionally lose your temper with your loved one. Instead, pick yourself up,

remind yourself of how much you love this person, and try harder next time to get things right. Don't hang on to any given incident. These only have instructional value. You can learn from them about what sets your loved one off and is likely to result on a meltdown. This will only hold back the progress being made in other areas. You're not a saint and you're going to screw up. Accepting this allows you to focus on what's important – supporting your Asperger's love one.

9. **Keep it Simple.** Don't try too hard to push your point of view on your loved one. People with Asperger's Syndrome sometimes have routines that make them feel safe; favorite things and places that provide a sense of belonging. Cultivate this tendency by not insisting that the routine that provides such comfort to AS people be deviated from. Instead, provide your full support for your AS loved one's need for regularity, predictability and routine. If you genuinely need to make a change, let your loved one know in advance. Carefully explain why (just this one time), you need some help re-organizing a particular day for a particular reason. Enlist your loved one's help in doing this. Involvement in an unexpected change to the daily routine of an AS person makes it much less confusing and difficult to absorb, as does careful reasoning about why the change is being made. Make sure you check that your AS loved one has put his car keys, wallet, book in progress and other important items in a consistent location. They won't do this on their own and not knowing where it is can result in scenes like the ones I witnessed in my life with Kendall. To avoid them, pick up the item when you see it in the wrong location and put it where it's supposed to be. This make life much more pleasant.

10. **Be realistic.** Don't expect to accomplish landmarks within an inappropriately specific timeframe (e.g., helping him find a full-time job at the age of twenty). Accept that there will be

hitches along the way, and that the goals you set at the start of your journey (at diagnosis) may not all be met. Sit down with your loved one and come up with a list of achievable goals, both long term and short term. The mutuality of the process, it's analytical nature and the sense of accomplishment it can provide an AS person will provide an important learning process for both of you and enhanced confidence for your loved one. I pursued this activity in a much more haphazard way with Kendall. While we'd discuss his symptoms in the aftermath of an outburst, or with regard to some of his other behaviors, presenting my viewpoint was illuminating for him. He'd often laugh at his own foibles when he was presented with the perspective of others in confrontation of the way he sometimes behaved.

11. **AS Children and Youth – Both Parents Need to be On Board.** This includes treatment, therapy, and rules you need to lay down for your child. Attend classes or conferences together which help you understand and learn more about Asperger's Syndrome and how to help your child or youth develop their life skills, while managing the condition. Talk openly about your child or youth's challenges and brainstorm possible ways for dealing with these as a team. Ask for outside help if needed, like signing up for couple's therapy. Couples with an Asperger's child have an advantage, as they automatically have a partner that can help with the many challenges of raising and supporting a child or youth with the condition. You're stronger as a team, but to be a team, you need to touch base with each other every day and be fully on board, as a couple. Imagine how much easier Kendall's life might have been had he been diagnosed as a child or youth. Imagine if his father had been diagnosed and he'd been prepared for a son with Asperger's? Their worlds would have been very different.

12. **Seek Out a Supportive Learning Environment.** Look for a learning environment that caters to and supports your child's special needs. Sometimes, if you have the resources, private school can be advantageous, but many public schools are equipped for special needs intake and should be investigated. Not everyone can afford to send a child to private school. If you're going to take the community school option, then arrange, with the rest of the family, to investigate the school's record with special needs children and youth, its principles, and especially, its record with AS students. Some public schools even have Additional resources for groups of special needs students and educational assistants expressly trained to work with them. You can find out where these are by checking in with the local Asperger's resource people, your clinician, or even the local Board of Education, or School District.

13. **Discuss the Condition with Your AS Loved One.** Your loved one needs to understand why being AS is so different, and why the perceptions of others can be difficult to absorb. This is especially important for teenagers with Asperger's Syndrome, since they feel the most pressure to conform to societal norms in order to fit in with their peer group. To help your loved one accept the condition and adjust to its challenges, it's important that you provide a basic understanding of what AS entails and why it produces the symptoms it does. Understanding leads to acceptance, which leads to people with AS arriving at an enhanced knowledge of the symptoms, behaviors, potential for those talents and gifts the condition can be home to and the potential for spinning these into a successful career, tailor made for AS people. Knowing this will help your love one find the right niche, and be more successful in life, as adulthood arrives. Kendall was lucky, in that life had led him to an ideal vocation to match his condition. Information Technology is a wonderful career for Aspies like him, but finding it was an

accident. That discovery also did not mitigate the impact of some of his disruptive behavior in the workplace, or his odd style of social interaction. These were responsible for his losing more than one job, even though Kendall didn't believe it. I watched it happen.

14. **Make use of Alternative Means of Communication.** A person with Asperger's Syndrome may find it easier to read notes or lists instead of communicating directly with people. While AS people should be encouraged to participate in social activities and to get to know other people, there should also be communication alternatives to direct, face to face interaction. This practice will accommodate the general AS need to step away from the loud, confusing world and into the internal one so well-loved by AS people. Consider the use of lists posted on the refrigerator door or cupboard, text messages, and e-mails. You can even go the extra mile and make tiny notes on post-its or small pieces of paper and place them in strategic places around the house in which your AS loved one will know to look for them. This practice ADHDs a level of intimacy to your relationship with your AS loved one. You have a secret message system that makes the condition easier to deal with when the time comes for withdrawal into AS's private world. I also found, with Kendall, that emailing a request (like groceries I wanted him to pick up) was easier than asking him directly. AS people are easily drawn into their own thoughts and away from the world that confronts them, especially when it becomes too demanding, or varied. An email will get their attention, especially if they're glued to their computer or mobile devices, as so many are, these days.

15. **Learn When to Walk Away.** A person with Asperger's Syndrome has very little interest in taking note of non-verbal cues and facial expressions. Sometimes, as I found with Kendall, this means they will be listening their internal

thoughts and miss what you're saying. You should pay careful attention to facial expressions while speaking to an AS loved one. If they look like they're not listening, or zoning out, they probably are. This means your AS loved one may miss important clues about your mood or state of wellbeing. Unlike other people, AS people don't read furrowed brows, angry glares and the slamming of doors in the same way. They won't respond to a kick under the tabling signaling that it's time to be quiet, while in a public place. These are clues not well absorbed by AS people. It can be really frustrating, especially in social situations. I remember many occasions on which I attempted to get Kendall's attention with non-verbal cues and failed. I was unable to head off intemperate comments and socially awkward behavior, because of this.

If you feel that you're experiencing an emotion that may lead to an outburst from one or the other of you, it's best to walk away, saying you've remembered there's something you need to do. Walking away from a potential conflict defuses it and also sends the message that you're unwilling to engage. If your AS loved one has missed a verbal cue, it may also have the effect of signaling that you have something to say, privately. While this won't immediately register, walking away will give you the opportunity to tell your AS loved one, directly, that he needs to adjust his conversation, attempts at humor, or even slow down his alcohol consumption, if you're in a social setting. This is also an exemplary behavior your AS loved one will learn from you, as a life skill to use in those moments when a meltdown is impending at an inopportune time. Walking away can head off a multitude of ills.

16. **Practice Good Hygiene.** A clean and healthy appearance can help boost the morale and confidence of your loved one. By instilling good hygiene habits, your loved one will have greater confidence to interact other people, whether in school, the office, or in social circles. Pay attention to clothing, as well and make sure your loved is wearing clothes that send the message

he's part of the world at the moment. That means actively discouraging your loved from clinging to clothing that's no longer in style. Worse, AS people have an unfortunate tendency to hang on to clothing items that have seen better days. Kendall had a favorite shirt that had seen better days. Toward the end of its long life I tried, many times, to stop him from leaving the house for work in this shirt. Finally, I threw it away. He was not happy, but there is nothing sadder than the sight of man wearing a shirt with the imprint of a hot iron in the middle of the back of it. There is an emotional attachment to such items for some AS people and your loved one should be encouraged to give away or discard them. Explain why you want them to do this in clear and simple terms. If that doesn't work, do what I did and chuck it. The argument will give you an opportunity to reinforce your loved one's understanding that other people don't get why wearing clothing that's torn, missing buttons, or bear the imprints of hot irons, is something your loved one gets a kick out of. While this may be embarrassing, your loved one will be given something to think about the next time a tattered clothing remnant looks like the right choice for a Monday morning.

17. **Introduce Your AS Loved One to Fun and Productive Activities.** A person with Asperger's Syndrome is most at ease when engaged in an activity that is of genuine (even obsessive) interest. This is more than a symptom. This is the root of the future and the realization of the AS person's peculiar propensity for prolonged and intense focus. Support your AS loved one in the pursuit of these interests and suggest others that might be of interest. Activities that interest you both are optimum, as they provide a site for bonding and sharing of your AS loved one's interest. This allows your loved one to regale you with the finer points of the interest and invite you into a world you may not always have such ready access to. Whether that's a trip

to the zoo (an interest in animals), the science center (physics and other scientific phenomena), or a sports match (statistics from the inception of whatever sport is concerned), an activity you can both enjoy, or include the entire family in, will boost your loved one's sense of belonging. It will also provide a setting in which you can deepen family relationships. Group activities are also recommended, particularly those involving music and art (if these are interests). Science, math and debate clubs are also great outlets for your AS loved one's fascination with details, analysis and language. Kendall enjoyed films and going out to eat different foods. He also enjoyed religious services we could both attend and learn from, as this was one of his pet topics.

18. **Keep Your Loved One's Neuro-psych Evaluations Current.** Neuro-psych re-evaluations should be done every three years, whether you think that your loved one's condition is improving, worsening, or unchanging. This is an important appointment to keep, to not only track your loved one's progress, but also to provide needed documentation in order to secure services for your loved one with Asperger's Syndrome (including education plans and medical benefits). Keep up to date with this and make a point of maintaining a schedule for these crucial appointments. A lapse can result in the loss of important services that benefit your loved one. To this day, I wish I'd been more insistent on clinical support for Kendall.

19. **Involve Your Loved One with Other AS People.** Whether it is a support group for people with Asperger's Syndrome, or just a group of individuals who share the same interests, it will be good for your loved one to be exposed to other people who live with AS. Instead of being the odd one out, being among others who struggle with AS will enable sharing and support, as well as acceptance. For example, if your loved one is interested in backgammon, you can look for a local backgammon club and

encourage attendance at their weekly (or monthly) sessions. Not only will it improve the expertise and knowledge your loved one has about the activity, exposure to other people who share the same interest will be helpful. Like-minded people will also enjoy the possibly obsessive interest your AS loved on has in backgammon (if that's the area of interest, but this applies to any interest in play). It's still important to remember that being around too many people who have the same condition as your loved one can also lead to meltdowns. A bunch of AS people in the same room, all speaking in the unusual way they do, can be a trigger, if the situation stresses your loved one out. There is the danger of over-stimulation, but this can occur in numerous settings. Look for groups in settings your loved one will enjoy optimum comfort, in order to boost confidence and social skills. You may have to try several groups or activities before you find the right fit, but that will be an interesting process for both you and your loved one. Ultimately, being in the presence of AS sufferers, or just others with the same interests will be a life enhancement.

20. **Side by Side is Better Than Face to Face.** A person with Asperger's Syndrome may be uncomfortable speaking to others face to face. The tendency of AS people is to avoid eye contact, as it may be interpreted as confrontational. Try talking to your loved one while walking down the street, or driving in your car, or eating next to one another, at meal times. Your AS loved one may find it more comfortable to engage in conversations without having to look at you, directly. This is especially important if you wish to speak with your loved one about something important. This simple communication hack can make all the difference in the relationship the two of you share. The level of comfort it will provoke will put your loved one at ease and that will be appreciated and make communication less difficult. In writing this, I recall that the

configuration of our living room contributed to Kendall's propensity for confrontation. We had two couches placed opposite each and each of us would sit on one of them. When I deliberately reconfigure the furniture to create a more open effect, placing the seat at the edges of the room, opportunities for confrontation were fewer and life at home more peaceful when we were both relaxing in the living room.

As helpful as these tips are, the bottom line is still this: you should make your own strategic plan—with the consultation of professionals and people you trust, of course—on how best to deal with a loved one with Asperger's Syndrome. Remember, above all, that patience is the key to successfully living with people with Asperger's, and in so doing, contributing to their success at living with the condition. Asperger's isn't an impossible condition. With patience, love, professional support and some planning, you and your AS loved one can lead happy, fulfilling lives together and in the world around you.

I wish things could have turned out differently for Kendall and I, but without the knowledge and support I needed, there was little I could do to change the outcome. Today, Kendall is an independent consultant, no longer subject to office politics, or the ability to "fit in" with people who don't understand him. By keeping his contact with the workplace to a minimum and interacting with clients remotely, or at intermittent meetings, he's enabled to engross him in the work he's so good at, while avoiding situations that can trigger outbursts, social awkwardness and job loss. This is a happy and workable situation for many AS people and it's made all the difference in his life.

CHAPTER 3

ADHD: DEFINITION AND TYPES

What is ADHD?

Attention Deficit Disorder, or ADD, is an outdated term for ADHD, and is now rarely used in clinical records. For the purpose of this book, I will treat ADD and ADHD as one and the same, and employ the acronym ADHD to describe the condition.

ADHD stands for Attention Deficit Hyperactivity Disorder, a neurodevelopmental psychiatric disorder most common in children, but also present in adults. In the USA, about 4% of adults are estimated to have ADHD. The condition is most commonly found in males, with an increased risk of more than 50% in male children. According to the CDC (Centers for Disease Control and Prevention), an estimated 6.4 million children have ADHD in the United States alone, making it one of the most common childhood disorders in the country. The rate of diagnosis increases at approximately 3% per year.

The CDC states that there is no known cause for ADHD, but that research has revealed a genetic link. A recent study, in particular, which examined the genetic makeup of twins found strong evidence to suggest a causal link in the genes.

Possible causes examined in the pursuit of more fully understanding the condition include exposure to environmental toxins. Lead is the substance researchers are most interested in this point. Brain injury is also a possible cause, as well as anomalies in vitro, leading to low birth weight, premature delivery and alcohol and tobacco use.

While none of these factors may be the actual, sole cause of ADHD, scientists believe that they represent risk factors for the development of the condition.

Schools of thought around the causes of ADHD include some unsubstantiated assertions that sugar consumption can lead to the condition. Causes cited by those seeking a trigger for the development of the condition include obsessive television viewing, difficult family situations and living in poverty. Science does not support any of these assertions.

While a great deal has been learned about ADHD in children, ADHD in adulthood is less well understood, as many who have the condition have never been diagnosed. This is particularly true of older populations. The same difficulties encountered by children with ADHD continue into adulthood, it's known. Therefore, the presence of an undiagnosed population represents something of a public health problem. Imagine that child in the 1950s or 60s, well before knowledge of the condition was widely diffused, would go undiagnosed, growing into an adult with all the same difficulties. These are symptoms the ADHD adult takes into the workplace, creating chaos there and at home. This can mean trouble securing and maintaining employment, making friends and forging romantic relationships.

Symptoms and Behaviors – Children with ADHD

Many children can get fidgety when asked to sit in one place for long periods of time. Kids are easily distracted and curious, so it's no surprise that a common childhood habit is forgetting to do those things they'd rather not – like homework. But ADHD children have a unique set of challenges in addition to being young humans (which can be tough enough).

There are three primary manifestations of the condition ADHD children may present, together, or in combination with others:

- Inattention (without impulsivity or hyperactivity).

- Hyperactivity and impulsivity (but attentive).

- Inattention, hyperactivity and impulsivity, in concert.

The final bullet point, above, is the one which describes the most common manifestation of ADHD and the most recognizable one, also.

Inattention

Children who feature the inattention associated with ADHD can fly under the radar and this can have some serious consequences for learning outcomes. While the inattentive ADHD child is gazing off into space, the learning cycle is going on apace. Inattention can also lead ADHD children to be out of step with the requirements of teachers and parents, due to not following instructions. Other children will wonder by their peer doesn't seem to play by the rules. It's hard to play by rules when you weren't paying attention while someone was telling you what those were.

Because of the subtler symptomatic manifestation of inattention in ADHD children, it's important to look out for the signs. Children who struggle with this characteristic tend not to pay attention to the finer points of various things (rules, for example) and are often careless about the execution of schoolwork. Easily distracted from the task at hand, these children can have difficulty focusing on and completing what they've been asked to do. Inattention can also leader to daydreaming and distractedness, presenting as detachment from the immediate environment. Inattentive ADHD children will also find it difficult to plan, organized and complete longer term projects, losing interest before they're finished them. They get bored easily. They lose personal items frequently, also.

The challenges of hyperactivity and impulsivity are much easier to detect. They tend to be disruptive in classroom settings, especially.

This can make life for educators difficult and impact learning outcomes for other children.

Hyperactivity/Impulsivity

These characteristics of ADHD are much easier to spot. Physical manifestations generally and those of the hyperactive/impulsive ADHD child are reasonably obvious, even in comparison to other children, who are generally active little creatures.

The hyperactive/impulsive ADHD child is always in motion. Veering from one activity to the next, they often leave partially completed homework in their wake, as they move on to the next item of interest that catches their busy eye. When asked to remain seated for any length of time, the ADHD child who presents these characteristics of the condition will be moving something, unable to stay still. A jiggling leg, drumming fingers, or bobbling up and down are all signs of ADHD hyperactivity/impulsivity.

The normal frenetic activity of young children is magnified in the hyperactive/impulsive ADHD child, who is constantly in motion, in one way or another, fidgeting in protests at being asked to remain in one place. Sometimes, the pressure of being in one place is too much for these children, and so they'll leave their seats at inopportune times, disrupting other children in classroom setting. There's also a tendency to talk constantly, which is another way these children are known to relief the pressure of being in social, or learning settings. Rarely will a child modelling these characteristics of the condition be seen as relaxed, quiet or even stationary. An unfortunate manifestation of hyperactivity/impulsivity is a quick temper when things don't go the way the child wants, or when the pressure of public settings becomes too much for them. They tend to "go off". Generally, these children can be difficult to manage in classrooms, as their constant motion and chatter distracts those around them.

Symptoms and Behaviors – Adults with ADHD

Adults with ADHD, whether diagnosed or not, can have a difficult time navigating social and workplace situations, due to their unique way of being in the world. If you believe an adult loved is displaying any of these symptoms or behaviors, it's important that you do your utmost to obtain a diagnosis. Adult ADHD is manageable, when the person with the condition and that person's family, social and professional network understand what's going on. Not knowing that can make life extraordinarily difficult for people with this condition. Job loss, broken relationships and social isolation can be avoided with a little knowledge and understanding. The icing on the cake is, of course, a diagnosis and therapy.

Adults with the condition are recognizable by a combination of behaviors. Some of these have to do with driving. A history of speeding tickets, inattention at the wheel and traffic accidents are some of the unfortunate results of ADHD adults taking to the road. This can mean the loss of a driver's license. An old friend of mine actually had her car impounded for a year. Not only had she racked up a pile of speeding tickets. She had failed to pay them. For many ADHD sufferers, this can be a recurring life problem, preventing them from working, due to the fact they are prohibited from driving.

Another hallmark of adult ADHD is a persistent problem with romantic relationships. In the context of a marriage, the condition can prove disastrous. But troubled marriages are common. Not everyone who's having marital difficulties is a candidate for a diagnosis. As stated above, though, undiagnosed ADHD can be minefield. A person married to an adult with ADHD can misinterpret inattention and a lack of follow through as not caring about the relationships. The tendency to be argumentative and temperamental are also difficult romantic partners to deal with, leading to discord and instability.

Poor listening skills and the tendency to go off into a private world of daydreams is another sign of adult ADHD. This can lead to problems at work, should the person drift off in meetings. ADHD adults are known to be inattentive to what others are saying and this extends to their romantic relationships and friendships, which can become strained because of it.

Procrastination is another serious problem for ADHD people. As with my friend who failed to pay her parking tickets, it's not that she didn't want to. She just kept putting it off until it was too late and the authorities caught up with her. Adult ADHD people are notorious, also, for failing to file their taxes on time, which can be the cause of major problems with the federal government, as years of unfiled returns catch up with them.

Hyperactivity/impulsivity manifests in adults with the condition as an inability to relax at appropriate times and difficulty sleeping. When this problem is persistent and long term, the result is that ADHD adults fall asleep at inappropriate times, as the fatigue this can engender catches up. Habits like leg shaking, nail-biting and stuttering can also be manifestations of this aspect of the disorder.

Needless to say, adults with ADHD face a unique set of challenges, as they attempt to maintain commitments to work, loved ones and relationships. When undiagnosed, life for ADHD adults can be a rollercoaster, twisting and turning through life's ups and downs chaotically and often, disastrously. Seeking a diagnosis for yourself or a loved one with the condition, is crucial. ADHD is highly responsive to many therapeutic strategies, which we'll discuss below.

While I've outlined some common symptoms and behaviors seen in children and adults with ADHD above, there are a number of clinical designations arising which can make therapy easier to apply. By recognizing this second layer of ADHD characteristics and specifically naming them, those with the condition are offered even more hope of managing their symptoms.

Types of ADHD

There are seven known types of ADHD, and the treatment for each one is different. A closer study of the symptoms should help determine which type is present in patients seeking diagnosis, and which treatment is best for each patient.

Following are the seven types of ADHD and their descriptions, as well as suggested treatments for them:

1. Classic ADHD. This type of ADHD is the easiest to diagnose and also the easiest to treat. The condition usually stems from low levels of dopamine in the brain. Symptoms include inattentiveness and hyperactivity. A child with classic ADHD also has difficulty concentrating on one thing and is easily distracted by other factors in the surrounding environment. ADHD people also have the tendency to be impulsive and disorganized. This can include a complete lack of interest in putting away clothing, tools and other items. Impulsivity can lead to displays of temper, hasty decisions, blurting out inappropriate thoughts and sudden shifts that make it difficult to complete tasks in progress. To help people with classic ADHD improve focus, stimulating supplements like green tea and ginseng can be helpful. You can also encourage physical activities, since these raise the levels of dopamine in the body and expend at least some of the impulsive energy ADHD people struggle with.

2. Inattentive ADHD. Similar to classic ADHD, inattentive ADHD causes a short attention span and procrastination. More often present in young girls than boys, inattentive ADHD also features significant introversion, which is accompanied by daydreaming and self-isolation. People with IADHD are easily distracted by little things, which can cause them to drop what they're doing and walk off in pursuit of another

interest. Unlike classic ADHD people, those with Inattentive ADHD are not hyperactive. Treatment for this type of ADHD is also focused on increasing dopamine levels, so a healthy diet, regular exercise, coupled with supplements that boost dopamine levels in the brain should help. This is discussed in detail in future chapters and will help you understand what you need to do for your child to boost their dopamine levels and get these to normalize, over time.

3.   Over-focused ADHD. This is polar opposite of Inattentive ADHD. Over-focused ADHD causes excessive focus on only one thing, at the expense of all others, causing Over-Focused ADHD people to have difficulty shifting their attention to other tasks and interests. This causes behavioral problems, especially if when being asked to shift focus by a teacher, parent, co-worker, or superior. Over-focused ADHD also precludes flexibility and adaptability, causing sufferer to be excessively reluctant to move from one thing to the next. The frustration at having to re-focus can be disruptive and interfere with daily life. Acting out is common. To help a person with Over-focused ADHD, try to avoid high-protein foods, because these can cause the patient to be ill-tempered. Over-focused ADHD people also need increased serotonin levels (as these are low in those who suffer with this variety of ADHD). Supplements such as saffron and inositol can be helpful as means of raising these.

4.   Temporal Lobe ADHD. Abnormalities in the temporal lobe may cause a people to have problems with memory and learning skills, as well as mood stability. This results rapidly realized irritability, and learning impairment. The impact of both short and long term memory loss or dysfunction can be manifested frustration and outbursts. To treat this type of ADHD, try administering magnesium supplements to help decrease anxiety and irritability. Gingko supplements can help

enhance memory and learning skills.

5. Limbic ADHD. Often misdiagnosed as depression, Limbic ADHD is actually caused by too much activity in the mood control center of the brain. Symptoms include mood instability, low self-esteem, feelings of guilt or anxiety, and a perpetual state of sadness. A diet rich in fish oil will help Limbic ADHD sufferers manage symptoms more effectively. Medication like Wellbutrin can also help, but make sure this is administered only under the supervision of a medical professional.

6. Ring Fire ADHD. Dubbed Ring Fire because of the images that appear in brain scans—like a ring of hyperactivity surrounding the brain—Ring Fire ADHD causes extreme, almost manic, hyperactivity. Episodes of meanness and unpredictability are common, as well as anxiety and irrational fear. Children with Ring Fire ADHD also suffer from extreme sensitivity, making them sensitive to light, noise, and human contact. To help a child with this type of ADHD, you can start with an elimination diet, to find out if an allergy is causing some of the symptoms. Once this possibility has been ruled out, supplements and medication can be administered under medical supervision.

7. Anxious ADHD. Aside from the usual ADHD symptoms (inattentiveness and distractibility) people with Anxious ADHD suffer from undue tension and anxiety. AADHD people may become unduly worried and anxious in social interactions, especially in those in which other people may judge the sufferer's symptoms and read them as social dysfunction. This may cause psychosomatic pain as evidenced by headaches, stomach cramps, and sweaty hands. Calming supplements like magnesium and holy basil can help your AADHD loved one reduce these symptoms. These supplements, in concert with antidepressants (administered only under medical supervision) and other medications can help boost dopamine levels, also.

CHAPTER 4

LIVING WITH ADHD

L iving with people with ADHD, whether children or adults, can often be a frustrating and exhausting experience. Classic ADHD causes those with the condition to be hyperactive and more often than not, unaware that their hyperactivity is disruptive and distressing for those around them. ADHD sufferers have no consciousness of these considerations.

Again, patience is the best tool in your tool box to help you live with a loved one who has ADHD, but patience is not enough. Following are seven tips you can call on to help you cope with living with a loved one with ADHD:

1. **Stay positive.** Don't be discouraged if you're not seeing progress from your loved one, despite all the treatment, medication, or therapy you're providing. Keeping in mind that people with ADHD are unaware of the effect their symptoms can have on those around them will help you maintain your cool, when the going gets difficult. This is especially true for children with the condition, as they can become very driven and single minded when they've set their hearts on a goal. Most children share this trait, but in ADHD children, it's quite extreme, which may sometimes come off as intentional misbehavior. Your focus should be on helping your loved cope with symptoms and managing the conditions, keeping in mind that applying the same rules you do to the non-ADHD world isn't going to work.

2. **Stick to a routine.** As with people with Asperger's Syndrome, people with ADHD function better in a setting governed by routine, including necessary tasks, organized into lists. This type of structure is very helpful to ADHD people. Planning the day in detail helps keep ADHD people on track, instead of wandering off course and falling prey to one of ADHD's primary challenges – the failure to follow through. This includes basic activities like eating, bathing, and sleeping, as well as more complex activities like homework, household chores, and playing outside the house, or other activities. When your ADHD loved one has a clear structure with suggested or necessary outcomes, the practice of focus will be more easily pursued. The frustration engendered by wandering off course and daydreaming can be replaced by the sense of accomplishment derived from meeting goals and the expectations of others.

3. **Manage with expectations.** Don't put a heavy burden on your loved one by expecting immediate or even steady behavioral improvements. Change is a long term project and ADHD's special challenges may require more time to improve, depending on the symptoms your loved one suffers from. Set ground rules that are reasonable and attainable. When setbacks occur, take them in stride. Take note of and learn from them. This practice will help you identify triggers that provoke certain behaviors in your loved one. In turn, understanding those triggers yourself can be a means of helping your loved one either avoid them, or understand how to assimilate them when they arise.

4. **Help your loved one make friends.** It may be hard for people with ADHD to build friendships because of the condition. The social impairment often exhibited by ADHD people can be difficult for those unfamiliar with the condition to understand. One way conversations and tactless statements, as well as

butting into the conversations of others can annoy other people when they don't understand where your loved one is coming from. The habit of "zoning out" when the subject of a conversation becomes boring is another disconcerting behavior that can lead to difficulties in social situations. Most people don't care to talk to someone who isn't listening, but this isn't understood by ADHD sufferers. Encourage your loved one to meet new people and make friends. Make sure to explain to new people in your loved one's life (or have your loved explain) what the situation is. People will be much more understanding when they're aware of the challenges presented by ADHD. They'll be less inclined to see your loved as rude, detached, or self-absorbed.

5. **Don't give up.** There will be times when living with ADHD will seem like the worst thing that ever happened to you. Life with ADHD can be a bit of a rollercoaster. Some days feel almost normal. Others seem like feeding time at the zoo. Be persistent and consistent. Stick to your guns. Don't let your ADHD loved one drift away from the schedule you've established. When this happens, reinforce its importance and value, with the same patience you always do. Try and try again, using other techniques that may be more effective if those you're using aren't working, depending on the situation. Remember: Your loved one needs your support and understanding, as well as your patience. This is a long term undertaking and you didn't get this far to bail now! Finish what you started and know that you're making a tremendous difference in the life of your loved one by agreeing to come along on this journey.

6. **Prioritize.** Don't try to get it all done in one go. This will only stress you out, as well as your support network (family and friends) and your loved one, most importantly. Determine which concerns need immediate attention, and deal with those

first. Take things one at a time and they'll seem less intimidating and much more doable. Temporarily set aside less important issues and tasks so you can focus on the most important ones. For example, if your child appears both socially awkward and depressed, you may want to deal with the depression first, before trying to move into the social aspects of ADHD. Depression can be a huge burden for ADHD people, but it's a common co-morbidity. If this is the case with your loved one, managing this aspect of the condition will lay a foundation for moving on to the social one.

7. **Educate yourself about ADHD.** Arming yourself with knowledge and experience, rather than charging into unknown territory, will prevent you from making mistakes that can hinder progress. Attend seminars about the condition, visit online forums and interact with other people who are fighting the same battles you are. Read books and magazines on the topic. The more you know about ADHD, the better you can strategize around living with it and the challenges it presents your loved one. However, be sure to consult reliable, accredited and professional sources which provide you with up to date, accurate information. It's easy to get lost in a sea of inaccurate information (especially online). Don't waste your time with sources that are less than reliable.

ADHD should not impede a child's growth, or ruin an adult's chances of enjoying long-lasting relationships, whether these are friendships, romantic interests, or professional associations. Whether your loved one is a seven-year-old child suffering from classic ADHD, or a thirty-two-year-old with Anxious ADHD, you can help by learning more about the condition, managing your expectations and being a steadfast support of living fully and well with the condition.

A Brief History of ADHD

ADHD is not a "new illness". It's been around for a while. Perhaps we now know more about it as an illness because of the modern willingness to be more open about disorders and conditions of this kind. Not so long ago, the stigma associated with mental health, personality and mood disorders was strong enough to keep discussion about them in the medical community. The public had little interest in considering the fact they might be living with these realities due to societal prohibitions and judgments about them, and the people who struggled with them. ADHD is a human reality that has always been with us, but has only recently been named and popularized for these reasons. This has opened the door to earlier diagnosis and more widespread acceptance.

Before the advent of medical specializations in mental health, people living with the wide spectrum of mental health challenges were left to the vagaries of an ignorant world. At the mercy of exorcists and superstitious judgments about the behaviors and symptoms they exhibited, they were socially outcast. Even today, there are places in the world where mental health challenges are viewed as aberrations to be locked away from prying eyes. In honor/shame cultures, mental illness or any kind of mental health challenge is feared for its power to bring shame to the families of sufferers.

In 1844, Heinrich Hoffman, a German doctor, was to produce a small book of illustrated stories intended to amuse his 3-year-old son, Carl Phillip. Included in the book was a chapter entitled "Zappelphillip" (Fidgety Phil), the story of a little boy who couldn't sit still. This story is now considered seminal to the development the medical profession's understanding of the condition. Today, it stands as the first illustration of what children with ADHD are like, particularly with respect to hyperactivity/impulsivity.

But ADHD was not identified as a clinical disorder in 1902. George Still, an English pediatrician, noted that there was a strong indication in some children to lack self-control. But this is not, by far, the full story.

In 1775, a physician decided to investigate what he believed to be an identifiable mental condition, and to observe a group of children who were all displaying similar characteristics. Adam Weikard documented the characteristics of the children in this control group. His explorations revealed that all children exhibited a propensity to self-isolate and refrain from interacting with the others in the group. These characteristics can also be seen in people with ADHD, as we now know.

Weikard's explorations also revealed that the children in his group preferred to remain busily occupied, but not necessarily in relation to other children in the group. He found that assigning tasks to these children was somewhat fruitless, as the group's children would rapidly lose interest in completing them, becoming distracted by something else that had caught their attention.

Weikard is said to have been assisted by Scottish physician, Alexander Crichton, who studied the yet unnamed condition in depth. Apart from observing and recording the behavior of these children, Crichton decided to study their mental condition. He observed that the children were not able to focus on any one thing for long periods and were easily distracted by what was going on around them. Everything from light, to heat and cold, to sounds caused these children to act out in protest at the change in environmental conditions. Crichton further observed that children outside the control group would not be affected to this extent. Finally, he noted the peculiar restlessness of children in the control group.

Apart child subjects of his observations, Crichton also observed adults who were known to have displayed similar symptoms in childhood.

These adults were also easily affected by distractions and had difficulty concentrating. Frequently, the adults observed by Crichton had significant challenges in maintaining employment, due to their lack of focus and failure to complete the tasks required by the day to day demands of their jobs.

Crichton was to publish the book, *Mental Derangement: Comprehending a Concise System of the Physiology and Pathology of the Human Mind,* detailing his findings in order to bring to attention to the importance that the condition be further investigated and treatments pursued, for both children and adults. The chapter of the book entitled "Attention" is the first attempt at a clinical description of the condition which would come to be known as ADHD.

As mentioned above, it wasn't until 1902 that George Still conducted further research into ADHD and came to the conclusion that the children he was studying must have been, at some point in their development, impacted by varying environmental factors which gave rise to their symptoms. Still was the first to content that there might be more in play than genetics, and suggest a developmental and/or environmental component.

But Still also attributed hereditary factors as key indicators in the likelihood that children would develop the condition. He believed the condition to be the result of both "nature" and "nurture". He also saw the condition as having positive aspects, as well as negative, due to his observation that the children involved in his research had the capacity to hold interesting conversations and boasted material analytical skills. In contrast, Still found that children deemed "normal" were not nearly so able to engage in conversations on advanced subjects and further, that they lacked the analytical capacity of the ADHD children. (Please note that using the term for the condition is an anachronism in this context, due to its not having been named at this point in history).

Over the two decades following Still's research, the condition began to be recognized with a much higher frequency in the general population. This led researchers to believe there was a genetic pattern at work. They believed this indicated that those who had ADHD as children passed it on to their own children, creating a generational chain. Research began to examine the genetic aspects of the condition. This included the identification of "hyperkinesis" (excessive activity) by German physicians, Franz Kramer and Hans Pollnow. They symptoms described in their 1932 report on the subject of hyperkinesis in children echo today's understanding of the manifestations of ADHD in hyperactive/impulsive ADHD children.

It wasn't until 1937, though, that an American physician discovered that stimulants had a beneficial effect on childhood symptoms of hyperactivity/impulsivity. Charles Bradley discovered that children at a home for childhood mental illness in Rhode Island, responded to this therapy. Today, these children would most likely be diagnosed as suffering from the condition.

Due to the prevalence of psychoanalysis as a panacea for the identifiable mental illnesses of the day, Bradley's findings weren't to be acted on for a further 25 years. But as time passed, more clinicians discovered the efficacy of stimulants like Benzedrine on symptoms. While this therapy is now discontinued for ADHD children and adults, stimulants continue to drive pharmaceutical therapy.

The use of Benzedrine was to be supplanted by the drug Methylphenidate, which was formulated by the pharmacist, Leandro Panizzon in 1944. The formula was later to be patented and marketed as Ritalin by Ciba-Geigy, in 1954. Today, Ritalin, while controversial, is a recognized pharmaceutical therapy for ADHD.

Ritalin, while having been seen to reduce ADHD's more disruptive symptoms, has controversial since its release. By the year 2001,

Ritalin by being prescribed to more than two million children American children each year. Dr. Nadine Lambert's report on the ongoing effects of the childhood use of Ritalin was cause for alarm for parents. Her findings pointed to an increased tendency for substance abuse (particularly amphetamines and tobacco), in adulthood. For example, Dr. Lambert found that fully 50% of children involved in her study were regular smokers by the age of seventeen. Another finding was that a small percentage of her sample became addicted to cocaine in adulthood.

Dr. Peter Breggin's report to the US House of Representatives' education subcommittee in 2001, also pointed to increased likelihood of adult substance abuse in children who took Ritalin. This, he found in his studies on the subject, was especially true of cocaine.

While other researchers and practitioners disagree that Ritalin use indicates later abuse of stimulants, not everyone agrees. By the same token the high profile controversy about Ritalin and its prescription to minor children, resulted in continued research which led to the development of other pharmaceutical options.

In 1996, the Federal Drug Administration approved the drug, Adderall. A psych stimulant, combing four amphetamine salts, this drug, while proving effective in the treatment of ADHD and narcolepsy, brings with it some unfortunate side effects, including social problems connected to its illicit and inappropriate use. College students, especially, have been known to abuse the drug in order to complete study assignments, by staying awake for long periods of time, using Adderall.

Many medical practitioners have sought to address this problem by switching patients to the new drug, Vyvanse, approved by the FDA for the treatment of ADHD in 2010. While successfully in treating ADHD with this alternative, it remains vulnerable to misuse as a study drug, in the same way that Ritalin and Adderall are.

In the late 80's the American Medical Journal identified ADHD as a separate and independent mental condition that affects both children and adults. This helped to spread awareness about it, leading to many children and adults finally receiving an accurate diagnosis and subsequent treatment.

As mentioned earlier in this book, the incidence of diagnosed ADHD is rising at a rate of 3% per year. Due to increased public consciousness and ongoing research, people who once fell between the diagnostic cracks are now being both diagnosed and treated. But this has not prevented ADHD from being a concern for parents worried about childhood diagnosis of the condition and what that meant for their children's continuing development and future success. It remains a source of parental concern, but also for continued research and study in order to find pharmaceutical solutions with fewer of the societal impacts drugs developed to date have proven to present.

In the late 80's the American Medical Journal identified ADHD as a separate and independent mental condition that affects both children and adults. This helped to spread awareness about it, leading to many children and adults finally receiving an accurate diagnosis and subsequent treatment.

Now, owing to public exposure and awareness about ADHD, more and more people are accepting it as a reality in their lives and coming forward with their stories. They are speaking about their own challenges, or on behalf of someone they know. The effect has been to lift the associated stigma and make life easier for people who live with the condition. Public understanding about ADHD and its effects on those who live with it has increased dramatically in recent years. Despite this new awareness, many continue to resist diagnosis due to self-stigmatization and cultural factors, as well the persistent ignorance about it in some quarters. Over time, it's hoped that awareness and understanding will encompass those who continue to suffer in silence because of these factors.

Treatments Prescribed for ADHD

We've now looked at the history of ADHD and also reviewed Asperger's Syndrome in some detail. It is understandably extremely difficult to be diagnosed with this condition. Whether diagnosis occurs in childhood or adulthood, it's not the easiest thing in the world to be told that you have another challenge to face in an already challenging life. ADHD is not untreatable, nor are its challenges insurmountable. They are, in fact, completely manageable with the right attitude, approach and therapy. Pharmaceutical medications, natural treatments and alternative therapies are all available for the treatment of ADHD. Combined with a healthy and positive attitude, the support of friends and family and sustained commitment to managing symptoms, people with ADHD can lead lives as successful and happy as anyone else.

We will look at all three of these in detail, starting with the pharmaceutical therapies. We'll look at what's available for children and adults. If you or a loved one has ADHD, it's incumbent upon me to remind you that whatever treatment you ultimately decide on, that this decision should be taken in conjunction with a professional medication consultation.

You doctor, once a diagnosis has been arrived at, will suggest one of the following types of medication:

- Stimulants

- Non stimulants

Stimulants

Stimulants are medicines administered for the purpose of increasing the production of certain chemicals in the brain and body. These chemicals work by affecting the part of the brain that deals with activity. Through the increased release of these beneficial chemicals it is possible for people with ADHD to control their hyperactivity. We've learned, at this point in our exploration, that children and adults who suffer from ADHD are afflicted with hyperactivity. This impedes their ability to stay in one place in order to focus long enough to complete study, work, reading and any other number of goals that need to be reached in their daily lives. By controlling the part of the brain that governs activity, it's possible for ADHD people to remain calm, focused and to remain in one place for longer periods of time. This enables them to concentrate on work and study and follow through on necessary tasks to completion.

Amphetamines are the most commonly employed pharmaceutical stimulant. This is, in fact, the drug most commonly used in the treatment of ADHD. The drug is given in varying dosages, depending on the age and symptomatic makeup of the patient. Amphetamines make it possible to increase the production dopamine, which is also known as the stress-busting hormone. This stimulant is preferred due to its rapid efficacy and for allowing people to consume it in two or three doses throughout the day. However, as good as this sounds, amphetamines come with several side effects. Patients may experience mood swings, dry mouth, headaches, migraines etc. So those who already have these conditions are advised to not take this medication and to seek alternatives.

As noted previously, Methylphenidates are the next most frequently prescribed treatment for ADHD, after amphetamines. These work differently than amphetamines and are considered alternatives for those seeking to avoid the side effects of the first alternative. But also have certain side effects.

As detailed in the section on the history of ADHD, science continues to examine new and better ways of medicating people with ADHD to help them manage their symptoms and behaviors more effectively. Also, the abuse of the three most prevalent pharmaceutical solutions to the condition, has led to much reflection in the scientific community about the cost of prescribing them to children. It's hoped that this research continues to render less risk to children who are prescribed medication for ADHD.

In either instance, a medical consultation is essential prior to pursuing a course of medication in the treatment of ADHD.

Non stimulants

Non-stimulants target other symptoms of ADHD and don't directly affect the brain. For this reasons, physicians prescribe them before prescribing stimulants. Their use is generally preferred, but in the event they don't work for the patient involved, stimulants are the next option. Non-stimulants are not addictive, which is a major selling point for both physicians and ADHD patients

Non-stimulants control blood pressure and help the address the patient's hyperactivity. By consuming non-stimulants, the patient will be able to conduct day-to-day activities without having to deal with disruptive or debilitating symptoms.

There are three types of non-stimulants prescribed for ADHD: Atomoxetine, Guanfacine and Clonidine. Each one has a different effect on the body and is prescribed in dosages dependent on the patient's age and activity level.

These also come with their fair share of side effects. They can cloud a person's cognitive functions, and cause dizziness. Adult patients may experience a reduction in libido and general energy level. If the patient begins developing sleeping problems and is unable to sleep at least 5 or 6 hours a night, then treatment is discontinued. This is important, as disrupted sleep patterns can aggravate the symptoms of ADHD. This can radically impact the success of treatment and the ability of the patient to function.

As is seen above, there are two distinct pharmaceutical options available for the treatment of ADHD and each of them comes with its own advantages and disadvantages. You can choose the type that suits your condition, age and body type. But remember that these medications are only available by prescription and under the advice of a physician. Seeking to treat yourself, or obtaining pharmaceutical through illegal channels can be dangerous to your health. Some of these products are expensive, but being insured and seeking discounted products can be done with the guidance of your medical practitioner and through your own investigations.

As with many pharmaceutical solutions, there is a danger of addiction to and abuse of stimulants. Young people prescribed ADHD medication have recently been seen to be selling or otherwise providing their medication to peers at exam time, or for simple amusement. This represents a significant risk to both patient and the peers to whom the medications are being provided. It's clear that amphetamines and other stimulants should only be administered under the care of a physician and not employed for simple amusement, or as a means of staying awake to completed assigned studies.

It's strongly counseled that the treatment of ADHD (whether yours, or that of a loved one) be closely monitored and guided by a medical professional. Should you fear that you or your love one is becoming addicted to the medication prescribed, consult your family physician at your earliest opportunity. There are other solutions that won't have this effect. You have enough challenges, as it is!

Natural Treatments for ADHD

In the previous chapter, we looked at the pharmaceutical medications prescribed for ADHD. Now, we'll look at natural therapies available to treat ADHD in children and adults.

Diet

Before we look at the natural supplements most frequently prescribed, we should first talk a look at the type of diet most effective for controlling the symptoms of ADHD.

To begin with, scrap junk and processed foods. These have no nutritional value and can be injurious to your overall health. Laden with preservatives, chemicals, salt, fat and sugar, junk and processed food doesn't do anyone any good. Our taste buds have been trained to crave them, from a life time of exposure. Marketing of these products (which can't really be referred to as food) exacerbates our cravings. Cutting them out of our diets is not what many of us want to do. It is, however, imperative, particularly if you or a loved suffers from ADHD. Start with this important deletion. Build a healthy diet that includes real food and not the highly processed rubbish that too often passes for food. It's also strongly encouraged that people with ADHD avoid foods high in sugar, as these can exacerbate existing hyperactivity and impulsivity. A stimulant which is helpful (for adults only, of course) is coffee. Adult ADHD people regularly report that drinking coffee balances their mood and mitigates symptom manifestation.

Fresh, seasonal food is a prescription for overall health. Fruit, vegetables, pulses, grains and beans are foundational foods that will be a great addition to the whole family's diet (if you're not eating much of them now). You'll all feel a difference and this is especially true of your ADHD loved one. A healthy diet which improves overall wellbeing is a good basis for addressing the challenges of the condition.

Nutritional content genuinely matters, so I'm including this handy reference to important nutrients your food should be providing to you, your family and your ADHD loved one.

Iron

Iron is an important nutrient, is essential for brain development and continuing health. It's vital eat food rich in iron, such as spinach and okra. Iron helps in improving cognition and keeps the brain alert and functioning optimally. A lack of iron causes sluggishness and inattention and can exacerbate the symptoms of ADHD.

Appropriate levels of iron in the body also help in increasing dopamine, which will slow down hyperactivity to a large extent. Great sources of iron include a bowl of cereal in the born, accompanied by fruit and full fat milk. Spinach soup and salads made with spinach is also a great way to increase the iron content of your family's daily diet. Iron is also present in red meat. While red meat is not something that should be a part of anyone's daily diet, eating this once per week can boost a system deficient in iron. Moderation, as with all things, is the key. Should you feel that your ADHD loved isn't getting enough iron in the daily diet, even with these iron hacks, then a supplement is indicated.

Zinc

Zinc is another important brain nutrient that can help improve alertness and energy. Zinc is needed to breakdown dopamine and transport it to the different parts of the brain. It is also known to work in tandem with iron to increase brain function and improve cognitive integrity. There are many foods rich in zinc, including oysters and beef. For vegetarians, wheat germ and spinach also contain high levels of the mineral. Toasted nuts and seeds make great, satisfying snacks and are very high in zinc. Again, a zinc supplement can work with the changes you're making in your loved one's diet, if you feel it's required.

Magnesium

Magnesium has an overall calming effect and can be especially helpful for people with ADHD, how are prone to outbursts and hyperactivity, as discussed earlier in this book. Foods rich in magnesium include green leafy vegetables like various kales and chards, dark chocolate and dried fruit. Incorporating these into the diet, as well as adding a supplement can make symptom management much easier for you, your family and your ADHD loved.

Omega 3

It is not secret that omega 3 fatty acids are essential for brain development and overall health. This is because they contain a chemical known as DHA, which is extremely important, especially for the developing brains of children. By incorporating this chemical in your loved one's diet, you will help in increasing his or her brain function. Fish is full of Omega 3 fatty acids and salmon or tuna are especially good, as they contain high levels of omega 3. For vegetarians, flax seeds are a good choice. They can be added in ground or powdered form to a variety of dishes, including salads or juices. You can also buy fish oil supplements for your child, available in health food stores and online.

Natural Treatment Supplements

Natural supplements are plant extracts administered to humans, because of their natural properties, known to humanity for perhaps thousands of years. These supplements are greatly preferred, as they don't tend to produce the side effects pharmaceutical medicines do. They are also easy on the body and don't negatively impact energy levels, due to their natural, unadulterated origins. Natural supplements are a great option for people with ADHD and can be used to supplement other therapies, including pharmaceuticals. They're safe to use, but if you're consuming a pharmaceutical medication, it's always best to check in with your practitioner to ensure there are no contra indications concerning combinations. Here are some of the best natural supplements for treating the symptoms of ADHD.

Ginseng

Ginseng is probably the most well known herb in the world. It is widely grown in China, where it's used for many purposes and recognized as a powerful agent of cognitive support. It's also said to increase brain function and physical vigor. Ginseng is a great herb to treat ADHD as it supports emotional control and will also help patients with concentration for study, work and other important tasks. Ginseng is available in tablet and capsule form. The raw herb may also be found in Chinese medicine outlets, as well as health food stores and can be made into a tea. In its raw form, Ginseng is said to be most effective.

Rhodiola rosea

Rhodiola rosea is a plant that is useful in treating ADHD. It is said to originate in the Arctic. You can buy it from a specialty shop or online. All you have to do is add the leaves and flowers to some boiling water, strain the boiled tea and cool it for consumption. You can also choose to administer tablets or capsules. Within a few months on this supplement, ADHD patients will show improvement, while remaining alert and active. This herbal remedy produces no fatigue and might also help people with ADHD develop better social skills, due to its effect in reducing anxiety.

Ashwagandha

Ashwagandha is a popular herb that is extensively used in traditional Indian medicine. The herb has powerful effects on the brain and is capable of both increasing cognition, while producing a calming effect that can help ADHD people with focus and hyperactivity. The herb has been used for many centuries to treat and also cure mental conditions and is sure to help reduce the symptoms of ADHD. Ashwagandha may be administered in tablet or capsule form, or bought as a powder, which can be dissolved in water and administered as a drink or tea.

Pycnogenol

This chemical is said to help the brain calm down and is helpful in producing increased powers of concentration. It is said to originate from trees found in France. The extract of the raw plant is full of anti-oxidants, which can help fight free radicals present in the brain, thereby reducing potential damage and even enhancing cognitive function. You can buy it from online stores or look for it at a specialty or health food store.

Shankpushpi

This is another herb grown extensively in India. The herb is administered to young children to increase their mental strength and clarity. You can buy the capsule or powder, which can be dissolved in water and administered as a beverage. You can also prepare a tea out of the leaves by boiling and distilling it. This herb is known to improve concentration and memory in those who consume it. Many Indian parents start giving this herb to their children just before an important test or exam to help improve their memory, enabling to be more adequately prepared and to excel. You can look for it in a traditional Indian food store or online. You can also buy Shankpushpi in syrup form for ease of administration.

Gingko Biloba

This is another globally popular Chinese herb used by millions for its effects on the brain. Gingko root is used to brew teas that help in reducing oxidative damage to the brain. ADHD patients will feel calm and relaxed and enjoy reduced hyperactivity and increased focus. Their cognition will improve and overall mental development will be enhanced, including concentration and focus.

With all the herbs and supplements listed above, it's important that you consult your family doctor before using them in your own treatment, or that of a loved one. While herbal remedies are natural, some of them may not be appropriate to combine with pharmaceutical therapies already in play.

Trial and error

Whether you're trying dietary changes or the supplements, you'll find there's a certain amount of trial and error involved. We're all different, which means that different things work for different ADHD patients. If one therapy doesn't produce the desired response, tweaks here and there and different combinations should be pursued until the you arrive at your goal. Elimination diets, in which certain foods, or therapies are eliminated one by one to gauge impact are also helpful in finding the right mix of therapies.

Alternative Therapies

As I said two chapters back, there are pharmaceutical medications, natural treatments and dietary therapies that work with the natural chemical makeup of your body to can help ADHD sufferers manage their symptoms more effectively. We looked at the first two types of supplemental therapies in the previous two chapters and in this one, we'll focus on the third type, being the alternative therapies.

As you know, when it comes to treating any form of illness, there's always a wide array of therapeutic choice available. This means you have the opportunity to either avoid pharmaceutical options (or reduce their dosage and thus, their impact on your body) and find natural remedies that can work for you. As previously stated, everyone's different and trying a variety of therapies is always advisable in a world of options. In this chapter, we'll look at some of the alternative therapies in existence that can work with other forms of therapy, or on their own, to help you or your loved one, manage the symptoms of ADHD.

Music

Music is the very first type of alternative therapy that you should consider in the quest for appropriate therapies for ADHD. Music is said to be a very powerful tool, which helps the human mind and body cope with almost any type of condition. It has been used to treat illnesses of varying degrees since time immemorial and has been found to help people challenged by all manner of mental and physical illness and injury.

Although taste in music differs from person to person, it's easy to understand that certain types of music are best suited and recommended, for people with mental health conditions. These types of music need to be calm and soothing and assist in transporting the person to a different world. It's safe to assume that classical music and also, soft instrumental compositions are particularly helpful. Music has an almost mythical curative power. Whether ADHD people choose to pursue music therapy privately, or to join a group that practices the therapy in community, the power of music is undeniable.

While effective for adults as well as children with ADHD, loved ones may find it difficult to present it to Aspies without encountering resistance. As with all therapeutic options, its necessary that your loved one be one board with availing themselves of any given therapy. It doesn't hurt to suggest, though! For children, though, music therapy is a solution that imparts important learning and support for the development of life skills and talents, as well as the social interaction so necessary for children with the condition.

While study continues into the effectiveness of this form of therapy, practitioners have found that applying music to the treatment of ADHD can result in the reduction of hyperactivity and impulsivity. They say that music sooths the savage best, so why not the beastly plague of perpetual motion, as experienced by people with ADHD?

The American Musical Therapy association recommends the pursuit of this strategy for symptom reduction through the application of a regular program, administered by accredited professionals. The therapy involves the use of music to encourage ADHD people to be more open about their emotional life and to help control their symptoms by being in touch with these. Music serve as a conduit for greater communication about the inner life of ADHD people, allowing them to connect behaviors and symptoms to their emotional lives.

Games

Many researchers have found that it is possible for children with ADHD to concentrate more effectively by encouraging them to play video games, where they're in control of the game, themselves. This is confidence builder, certainly, but it's important that electronic games not be relied upon as a therapeutic tool. Many children are glued to video games, which isolates them. For ADHD children, the effect can be to compound their sense of isolation, which represents a setback, as they already suffer from a certain degree of social isolation. For this reason, it's important that parents of ADHD children be aware of and limit the time their children spend playing video games. Much more useful is community play, especially involving other children.

Whether the ADHD sufferer in question is a child or an adult, the power of play is undeniable. We all need to reach outward, toward the fun in life. This be can be pursued in many ways. Children play naturally, but as we grow older, we lose our sense of play and whimsy. While some say that this is a part of adulthood, the limitations implicit are obvious. When life becomes burdensome, a little play (at any age) is advisable and even, an imperative.

Play is our soulful natures finding wonder and fun in the world around us. You can play with your ADHD loved one in many ways. If your loved one is a child, taking the time to pursue play as part of your weekly schedule, is highly advised. Play can involve riding bicycles, playing on the swings in the park, or throwing a ball around. There is nothing more wonderful for ADHD people than to be engaged in an activity that is "just for fun". Find the one that appeals to you and your ADHD loved on and go to town!

Adult play can be everything from skiing to geo-caching. Dancing is also a good one. ADHD people, particularly, may enjoy line dancing, due its demand that participants focus and act in unison with other people. This activity can impart a sense of belonging and accomplishment, as it demands the kind of focus ADHD people are famous for. With play, the sky's the limit. The world is full of fun, so let your imagination run wild and find the playful activity that invites the most enjoyment.

Games like backgammon are especially well suited to the analytical excellence of people with ADHD. They can see the next move well before you make it and delight in winning. This can become a little frustrating for we non-ADHD people, as it's tough to lose every game to our analytically superior ADHD peers! Another game ideally suited to people with ADHD is Scrabble, with its demand that players have a commanding grasp of the English language. ADHD people are known to have impressive vocabularies. Again, losing will suck, but the interaction with be fun for everyone involved. You can also try Trivial Pursuit, as trivia and its collation is a beloved pursuit of people with ADHD.

Yoga/ tai chi

Yoga is a traditional form of exercise that is practiced to find relief from mental and physical conditions and to strengthen the body and mind. There are many poses to choose from and you can choose those which promote relaxation and increased mental balance and calm. There are many Yoga classes available, but some forms of Yoga may be more beneficial for the condition in question than others. Take your time. Explore and find the one that's most effective for you, or your loved one.

The yogic practice of *pranayama* (breathing exercise) is a very good choice to help ease the symptoms of any of these conditions mentioned in this book, but may be especially suitable to ADHD people, due their centering function. Also, learning the bridge pose, pigeon pose, shoulder stand and headstand might be beneficial, depending on the severity and combination of symptoms in your case. In the case of a loved one, ensure that adequate supervision is provided and that the poses, or breathing exercises are being executed correctly, for maximum benefit.

Tai chi is another practice which can help ease hyperactivity and inattention, due to the slow deliberate movements followed. Tai chi classes can be found in many places. Check your local community center's calendar, or ask your medical practitioner.

Mirrors

Researchers have found that people with Asperger's, ADHD and autism can benefit from certain activities performed in front of a large mirror. The mirror provides the ADHD person with the opportunity to see themselves as others do. The use of the mirror offers a means by which people with these conditions can receive auto-feedback on methods for perform a variety of actions and also serve to remind them of the nature of their presence. This can provide a window into the perceptions of those around them and perhaps work to explain them to the person with the condition, at least to a degree. By allowing the person in the mirror to provide reinforcement and clues about the perceptions of others, the ADHD can become more conscious of the effects behaviors and symptoms in play on other people.

Especially for ADHD children (who may experience delayed development in terms of self-perception), a mirror can reinforce childhood development of the ability to perceive a distinct and unique self, by providing a model of third-party feedback, without the judgment inherent in that same feedback from actual third parties. In other words, mirror therapy provides a type of preview of the real world in a non-threatening, clinical environment.

Hobbies

A common thread running through all the conditions mentioned in this book is that of keen focus on one or several pet subjects, topics or interests. This characteristic can become a positive in the life of people with these conditions, with the addition of a hobby that can serve as an outlet.

Transforming obsession into a positive, productive hobby is a way to validate the less disruptive aspects of Asperger's, ADHD and autism, harnessing them to make them more welcome in the life of people who struggle with them. For either yourself, or your loved one, exploring your areas of interest and how you might make entertaining and life-affirming hobbies from them is an exercise in making lemons out of lemonade. What might be seen as an annoyance by many, can find a whole new definition in the pursuit of channeling an obsession into hobby that brings joy. Whether it's building models or robots, collecting stamps, painting, or reading, having an absorbing hobby is part of life people with these conditions can genuinely benefit from.

Sports

Taking part in sports activities is always a great outlet for the energetic hyperactivity these disorders tend to feature. Sports activities such as swimming and jogging, or playing a team sport like baseball, basketball, softball, football or tennis, will encourage relaxation. The physical activity will also boost the release of serotonin in the body, working to suppress the production of the natural depressant, cortisol. Pursuing a sports activity or team sport for one hour a day, five days a week, can be part of the schedule we've discussed earlier in this book. Like a hobby, it's something to look forward to and a great way for people with Asperger's, ADHD and autism to connect with other people in their peer and age groups.

Acupressure

Acupressure is another alternative therapy that can be explored in order to manage the symptoms of all the conditions discussed in this book. An acupressure therapist will be aware of the most advantageous parts of the body to work on and how these correspond to areas of the brain that govern certain responses, particularly those which generate symptomatic behaviors. Acupressure therapy can help in reducing hyperactivity, inattention and even depression. Take your time and seek out a licensed professional. Ask for recommendations from your support network.

Nature

Nature has a healing power for most people, but for those living with Asperger's, ADHD, or autism, it's power is multiplied. The presence of the natural world is a source of fascination, full as it is with plants, trees, insect and bird life. This can be a source of wonder for people with these conditions. Visiting parks, botanical gardens, or forests is an excuse to step out of your day to day life. Scheduling such visits can be a welcome departure from the day to day routine of your well-ordered life. But adding them to the schedule periodically, as gives you and your loved one something to look forward to, even if you're just going down the block to the park for a little play on the swings. (Adults need to play, too, remember?)

You can also bring nature into your home with the addition of indoor plants, or take to the garden (if you have one). Aquariums, insectariums and cacti can also be sources of intense fascination. Should you have a garden, you and your love one can choose plants to cultivate together, or start a container garden. Imagine the joy of eating things you've grown? Setting your own food on the table imparts a sense of accomplishment and pride. Maybe you, or your love one, are closet organic farmers?

Trekking and hiking regularly is a convenient way to combine exercise with exploration of the natural world, also. Climbing trees, discovering forests and enjoying all the natural world has to offer takes people out of themselves, while strengthening their bodies and reinforcing their health. This can be an icing on the cake in the therapeutic world of ADHD people; something fun and liberating that doesn't seem like work is always a welcome addition.

Pets

Pets can have a positive impact on the human psyche. The presence of an animal, whether a dog, cat, bird or hamster, provides a source of companionship and stewardship that is very supportive of symptom management. The sense of being necessary and having a purpose in the life of a creature also generates feelings of responsibility, through the provision of the routine care required. Adults and children alike will love to take care of their pet, which will increase their sense of responsibility and accountability. Whichever animal you consider adding to your family, the benefits of pet ownership for people with these conditions can't be overstated.

Animal therapy is also a growing area that provides effective, therapeutic support to people with the conditions this book discusses. Animals, unlike humans, offer people the unconditional love and acceptance many children and adults with spectrum conditions and ADHD so badly need. Autistic children and adults are particularly helped by the presence of animals, interacting with them and learning to care for them.

Equestrian therapy is becoming more and more popular, as it provides the opportunity for children and adults with these conditions to experience a large, powerful animal which is also specially trained to be gentle and sensitive with its human, special needs friends. The relationship between the rider and the horse, the rocking sensation encountered while riding, as well as the involvement of participants in the care, feeding and cleaning of horses, promotes greater confidence, motor skills and improved social awareness.

Finally, therapy animals which have been provided by a service which trains and grooms them as life supports to people with autism, Asperger's and ADHD, can be the best friend people with these conditions will ever have. The constant support of a trained therapy animal is proven to be beneficial in symptom reduction and coping skills. There are many organizations which train specialized therapy animals and match them with those who need them. There's most certainly one in your area.

Counseling

Professional counselling can provide people with the conditions we've discussed in this book a sounding board which reduces reliance on the input of caregivers and other members of the support group. It's highly advised that you seek out and avail yourself of this type of therapy. It will serve as a compliment to therapies being undertaken in the family and its support network. It will also provide a professional lens through which to view progress, setbacks and possible tweaks to therapies underway.

Group counselling may also be helpful for many people with Asperger's, ADHD, or autism. Placing yourself or your loved one in a setting with others who struggle with these conditions is a contextual shift, widening the world through the experiences of others with similar challenges. The effect is to make people with these conditions feel less alone in their struggles and also, less odd. Knowing you're not the only one is a powerful thing. Hearing stories like your own is an effective means of self-validation and acceptance, also. Your family physician or another clinician in your support network can guide you to either individual or group counselling, or you can check your local support organization, depending on you or your loved one's condition.

Intelligence

Children with Asperger's, ADHD are often highly intelligent. It has been observed that they boast enormous vocabularies and sometimes and impressive verbal facility. People with autism often have musical and artistic talent far beyond what might be imagined. Asperger's and ADHD people, with their intense analytical focus can be found working in fields like data management, information technology and statistical collation. These are uniquely suited to what might otherwise be considered an annoying and obsessive character.

The unique focus of people with these conditions renders them suitable for careers as scientists, inventors, and other vocations which demand a high degree of focus and detailed work. Some believe that geniuses like Albert Einstein and Sir Isaac Newton were ADHD people, but that instead of allowing it to push them off their life trajectories, they embraced their symptoms, choosing to employ their unique character traits in the service of humanity. But they're not alone in their status as famous people with ADHD. In our day and age, increased awareness of the condition has caused many celebrities and sports personalities to come forward as having been diagnosed with it. These include journalist Lisa Ling, actor Channing Tatum and superstar actor, singer and musician, Justin Timberlake. These people are living proof that people with ADHD can be successful or even world famous.

Creative nature

Creativity is a hallmark of all these conditions, depending on the combination of symptoms implicated and the severity of the disorder in play. People with these conditions have unique worldviews well-suited to creative pursuits and the creative solution of problems which may elude others. This creativity is to be cultivated by providing opportunities for people with Asperger's, ADHD and autism to nurture their creative gifts. Art, music, sculpture, physics, writing, film-making, even computer programming – the sky's the limit for the creative gifts of people living with these realities. They're special people with special gifts which can serve the world and make it more beautiful.

CHAPTER 5

AUTISM – DEFINITION AND TYPES

Of the three conditions this book focuses on, autism can easily be described as the most difficult to live with. While autism, being on a spectrum that encompasses everything from severe to relatively mild symptoms, its impact on the lives of those who live with it is material and sometimes, very difficult to cope with, indeed. Asperger's Syndrome (as discussed earlier) is part of the autism scale. The clinical name, Autism Spectrum Disorder, encompasses a diversity of symptoms and severity of those symptoms.

The CDC's statistics indicate that approximately 1 in 68 children in the USA is diagnosed as being on the autism scale. Over the past forty years, the prevalence of autism has increased exponentially and is now 10 times more likely to afflict American children. Far more common in male children, autism is said to found in 1 of 42 boys. With its frequency in girls estimated at 1 in 189, this disparity means that the likelihood of boys being diagnosed with autism is four or five times higher than it is for girls.

Autism is a societal reality that affects more than 3 million people in the United States alone and 10s of millions, all over the world. Globally, statistics kept by a variety of governments indicate that diagnoses of autism have increased by between 10 and 17% over the past several years.

The terms ASD and autism both refer to a cluster of disorders arising from the development of the infant brain. Symptoms include social impairment, as well as impairment of communication (both non-verbal and verbal). Repetitive movements, rigidly ritualized routine and an inability to sustain eye contact are also common symptoms. Some forms of autism are typified by impaired cognitive or intellectual function, problems with physical co-ordination and inattentiveness. There are often sleep and GI (gastro-intestinal tract issues with some forms of autism, as well.

Math, art and music are areas in which autistic people are often seen to display superior skill and talent, often in the presence of severe symptoms.

In the spring of 2013, the DSM-5 diagnostic manual (used by clinical professionals), moved to merge all disorders characterized by these symptoms onto what is now call the ASD scale. This changed the previous practice of defining all orders on the scale as unique from one another and distinct. Included on this scale are Asperger's, childhood disintegrative disorder, and pervasive developmental disorder.

Let's review the distinctive characteristics of each of these varieties of ASD (with the exception of Asperger's which has already been discussed at some length), as well as available therapeutic options for them.

Childhood Disintegrative Disorder

This ASD type is also known as Heller's Syndrome, or disintegrative psychosis. Some of its symptoms include delayed development in communication and social skills, as well as motor coordination.

Originally identified by Theodor Heller at the dawn of the 20th Century, its definition pre-dated the description of autism by Leo Kanner and Hans Asperger by 35 years. Heller's term to describe CDD was originally dementia infantilis (infantile dementia).

CDD sets itself apart on the ASD spectrum due to its unusual manifestation, which is typified by a regression from learned skills, or a loss thereof, usually occurring after a period of relatively normal development of approximately three years. Parents will note a dramatic change in the child's development, with the child also sometimes being aware that there has been an important change in their ability to what they have been able to, up to the point deterioration commences. The condition and its manifestation is sometimes accompanied by hallucinations. Incontinence (lack of control over bowel function, or bladder function, or both concurrently) is also a symptom.

It's sometimes the case that children who later present CDD already appear to be stalled or delayed in their development. Because not all children develop at the same rate, though, delays of this nature can be less than obvious. This form of autism, due to its insidiousness and odd manifestation, can be particularly difficult for children who have it, as well as their families.

Treatment of CDD is a subject of much controversy, as it is such a devastating form of autism. It is accepted, however, that this variety of autism doesn't respond well to the application of stimulants in its treatment. That said, there are some standard approaches to the treatment of CDD that offer hope.

Behavior therapy (also referred to as Applied Behavior Analysis, or ABA) is a therapy that attempts to re-establish skills the CDD child has lost. These include self-care life skills, communication and social skills. Rewards are used as a means of validating the desired behavior and to work with the child at eliminating undesirable behavior arising from CDD symptoms. Widely employed across numerous health care disciplines, from physical and speech therapists to psychologists, caregivers are included in the therapy and encouraged to consistently use its methodologies in the course of day to day life.

A second therapeutic strategy for CDD children is Environmental Therapy (also referred to as SET, or Sensory Enrichment Therapy). This therapy employs augmentation of the senses of the child, toward re-establishing a command of the senses (as this variety autism is less cognitive than sensory in its manifestation).

Pharmaceutical therapies for direct and specific treatment of CDD are not currently available, but the use of antipsychotics are sometimes used in the event that disruptive or harmful behavioral factors are in play.

Pervasive Developmental Disorder

PDD actually describes five distinct sub-types, featuring frustrated development in a spectrum of basic, human functioning. As with other disorders on the scale, these are most commonly recognized in delayed communication and social development. There is divergence as to some of these sub-types' inclusion on the autism scale, but clinical practitioners generally place them there, due to the symptomatic similarities inherent.

PDD most commonly manifests in infancy, but is very difficult to recognize and thus, diagnosis, until about the age of three. PDD is usually manifested in the slow achievement of a variety of developmental milestones, particular motor and communication skills. These are usually the first indications the sub-type noticed by parents of children with this type of autism.

The use of the appellation is controversial in itself, partially due to the fact that physicians are reluctant to arrive at a diagnosis in children who are still in the toddler stage of development. It's generally accepted, though, that PDD refers to a cluster of related varieties of autism and not to a unique, standalone disorder.

Diagnosis for this difficult to spot condition includes trouble understanding the relationship of the self to the objective world, as well as interacting with others. Lack of eye contact and the absence of facial animation also indicate this effect. Toys may be played with in ways that seem odd. A change in routine can result in a tantrum in children with PDD, due to their need for routine (common in many ASD spectrum conditions). PDD children also don't care to be touched by others and suffer from an inability to control their emotions. This can lead to aggression and tantrums. Some PDD children are complete non-verbal, while others have limited verbal ability. Others seem relatively normal in their level of linguistic development. Repetitive actions and poor social skills also are key indicators of PDD.

Therapeutic supports for PDD children are recommended to be highly individualized to the patient, due to the range of symptomatic manifestations in this variety of autism. Learning environments designed to accommodate children with PDD and similar ASD cousins involve limited classroom environments, hosting fewer students, and intensive support from specially trained educational assistants. The sooner PDD is diagnosed, the better the prospects for children with this condition. Early detection and diagnosis, followed by therapeutic intervention (particularly educational and clinical counselling solutions) are strongly advised.

No matter where a child (or an adult) falls on the autism spectrum, there's little doubt that no matter how manageable their symptoms may seem at first glance, these folks are different. They see and respond to the world so differently, that those with no knowledge of ASD can find them bizarre to interact with.

As with all the disorders discussed in this book, continuing education is leading to a greater understanding of autism and its implications for the people who live with it.

Next we'll explore some life tweaks caregivers can consider in the project of living with loved ones who have autism.

CHAPTER 6

LIVING WITH AUTISM – STRATEGIES AND THERAPIES

Part of the reason this section of the book is so important to me is my experience of autism. I've met many autistic people over the course of my life, but here I offer three examples of the wide variety of the experiences of autistic people in the world. These are all wildly different and reflect a shift for the better in societal attitudes toward autism and those who have it. They illustrating the changing status of people with autism and also the increased hope for managing their systems in greater public awareness and therapeutic answers. I hope they'll serve to illuminate aspects of the personal situation that led you to choose this book and provide a helpful look at the diversity of the autistic experience.

Ricki

I grew up in a small town in the 1960s. It was a conservative, parochial little place, surrounded by agriculture and nature. We rode our bicycles to school. We left our doors unlocked and roamed about at will, as kids. I'm lucky to have had the quintessentially idyllic childhood. But the naïve nature of the times was demonstrably responsible for the experience of people with autism. There was little support in those days for autistic people and little public understanding of the disorder.

In elementary school, I had a friend who was always a little different from the other kids at our school. Her name was Ricki and she was extravagantly and resolutely unusual. She marched to the beat of not only a different drummer, but an entire orchestra (apparently of intergalactic alien origins).

Some kids saw Ricki's unusual character traits as a license to pick on her and pick on her they did, with great gusto. Ricki's friends were few, but we were fiercely loyal. We instinctively knew she needed us to beat off the bullies. Ricki was a virtual bully magnet, attracting every maladjusted brat for miles around with her plucky "otherness". We didn't know quite where it came from, but we knew she wasn't like the rest of us is some intangible, fundamental way.

Many decades have passed and Ricki and I are still friends. I'm also friendly with her cousin, Susan, who was a high school sidekick of mine, years after my youthful experience of Ricki. It was at the time of return to my hometown to live for several years, that I re-connected with them both, to my delight. Ricki was still Ricki and Susan? Susan was utterly exasperated with antic behavior of her wacky cousin.

Frequently we would engage in long conversations about what do with a problem like Ricki. In adulthood, Ricki had married and divorced in short order, leaving her alone in the wilderness and to her sometimes unfortunate devices. Her life was a patchwork of disaster and triumph, which triumph was usually precipitated by the intervention of her longsuffering family, including Susan.

Ricki had a tendency to forge relationships with inappropriate men, suffering in the wake of the inevitable demise of these liaisons, usually a little financially and spiritually bruised by them. Ricki had a bad habit of zoning in on the most inappropriate men in her immediate sphere and latching onto them for dear life. She was a sucker for a pretty face and these guys knew it and took full advantage. There were tales of men insinuating themselves into her life and home and also tales of the financial toll the men in these tales took on my old friend. Unable to rationalize why she shouldn't be so ready to trust; Ricki has suffered in these situations throughout her life.

Family gatherings were often the site of anxiety and general dread for Susan, who couldn't, for the life of her, understand what in the hell was going on with her strange cousin. A sense of humor that set people's teeth on edge was something to be endured, regardless of the occasion. Demands for the most expensive booze on offer were blurted out the moment Ricki arrived to celebrate the occasion. Strangely timed outbursts of hilarity at inopportune times were the order of the day. These left Susan at the point of avoiding all contact with her cousin. But then it occurred to her something was missing in the great scheme of things. What was missing, in her estimation, was a diagnosis of some kind. She knew something more than an unusual personality was at work, and so she took steps to get Ricki to the doctor.

The straw that broke the camel's back was yet another job loss for Ricki. Her work at a local boutique had ended in tears and the usual recriminations and Susan was growing concerned for her cousin's future and her own sanity. The repetitive patterns of Ricki's life had been somewhat allowable earlier in her life. In her 50s, though, these were becoming life threatening. Susan feared that if someone didn't act and soon, that Ricki would become a statistic – homeless, alone and hungry, due to her apparent inability to fit in the way the rest of the world expected her to.

And that's when Ricki was diagnosed with autism. It changed everything.

Suddenly, Susan understood where Ricki's strange behaviors came from. The family that had long written her off as being intractable and irresponsible finally saw the writing on the wall and it said – ASD. Reflecting on my experience of Ricki early in life, I felt a sudden rush of compassion for a lonely little girl, who had never been diagnosed, left to wonder why it was so hard for her to get along with other people. That little girl had grown into an adult woman, uncertain why it was she couldn't seem to permanently latch on to anything or anyone in life.

Ricki was able to draw government disability because of her autism diagnosis. This ended the cyclical disappointments and devastation that had, until diagnosis, been the story of her life. Diagnosis also allowed Ricki to live quietly, pursuing her interests in art, history, music and dance. Her diagnosis so radically improved her life, I felt almost angry that no one had sought to seek a diagnosis before this point in her life.

But the thing with Ricki is that her symptoms weren't obvious. She was different, weird, inappropriate, reckless and odd. Nobody thought for a minute she might be autistic and then, her cousin took action. And the times we grew up in weren't designed to accommodate people with Ricki's diagnosis. Knowledge of the condition was limited and this caused a great deal of lost potential. The gifts of many autistic people have been lost to the world due our failure to more rigorously seek to understand it.

Ricki has a life now, entirely due to Susan's intervention. Her life has never been this full, rewarding and above all, fun.

Bob

Life in the Church exposes one to a wide-ranging experience of the human condition. There you'll meet everyone you could possibly imagine. From ex-cons to saints, to philanderers and floozies, the Church is a hospital for sinners seeking holiness and a riotous carnival of human foibles in the midst of sincere belief and genuine devotion.

It was during the course of my life as a church coordinator that I met Bob. The small urban parish I worked at was part of a cluster of parishes, clinging together in a world grown disinterested in religious practice for dear life and basic survival. Bob was from one of the other parishes, but regularly presented himself each Thursday morning to assist with the weekly luncheon for the area's poor.

I usually heard Bob coming before I saw him. He spoke in a loud monotone, usually peppered with detailed information about the cluster's various services and which of the priests would be presiding at each of them. Even if he'd already regaled other parishioners with this useful information in the narthex of the church, Bob would make a point of bursting into the office and regaling me with precisely the same information, at full volume.

"Use your inside voice, Bob!" I would say (at times impatiently). The church was a hectic place on Thursday mornings, with lunch guests (of all temperaments, life stations and states of mental health) popping in for a chin wag. Many came inordinately early to secure a seat and hang out with cronies who'd come from other parts of town for the popular, weekly event.

I would listen patiently for as long as time would allow, interjecting here and there to remind Bob that I actually typed the monthly worship rota, so I was already familiar with the information. That did not stop Bob. Bob did not care. I was going to hear it from beginning to end, or risk inducing his frustration.

Bob was in his 40s at the time and lived in a care facility run by the parish. His church activities formed the nucleus of his life. But perhaps Bob's favorite part of the week was his regularly and strictly scheduled visit to the local chicken restaurant, where he always ordered precisely the same meal, at the same time and ate it in precisely the same way, at the same table. This weekly event, like the church lunch, was Holy Writ. Like the recitation of the rota, not to be interrupted, or in any way interfered with.

Like Ricki, Bob was autistic, but with much more pronounced symptoms. His facial features also hinted at the condition and his expressions ranged from mild amusement to mild annoyance, but rarely deviated from these narrow manifestations of his frame of mind.

Famously, Bob was also known to disrupt church services on a regular basis, blurting out corrections to the liturgy, or repeating the words of the priest's sermons as it was delivered. A firm hand was needed at moments like these, as well as the unwavering patience of all the priests who ministered to the cluster. Bob's behavior sometimes drew the ire of a less than patient parishioner, but for the most part, people were accustomed to it. They knew Bob was autistic and loved him just the same, disruptions and all.

Context was also very important to Bob. Encountering me outside my normal context (the church office) was an unwelcome event. If we happened to meet on the bus, for example, Bob would have to be actively pressed to acknowledge me, preferring to pretend I wasn't there. I wasn't supposed to be there. I wasn't usually there, so it was easier for Bob to pretend I was not, in fact, there.

Bob's early diagnosis, a loving and patient family and an extended church family that cherished his presence made of his life a pleasant adventure. His love of detail and willingness to participate in all the cluster of parishes had to offer, gave him a profound purpose and days filled with things to do and lists to repeat. Bob is a lucky autistic gentleman, indeed.

Salvador

I've been fortunate to enjoy a life of variety and adventure which has included a great deal of travel. Mexico is a favorite destination of mine and the beautiful city of Puerto Vallarta, in the province of Jalisco, is a second home. The people of Mexico are predominantly friendly and welcoming toward those of us from other nations who vacation and live among them. An added bonus is that the city's status as an international resort destination has compelled many of the people who live there to acquire at least a conversational command of the English language. This makes it more difficult, perhaps, for English-speaking visitors to learn Spanish, but it also provides ample opportunity to get to know Mexicans on their own turf and on their own terms. Practicing English and learning to speak it well is a value in Puerto Vallarta.

Salvador is pre-teen boy, strongly built and tall for his age. His English is almost impossibly perfect, because Salvador was once blessed with the opportunity to participate in an educational exchange program that took him out of Mexico, to distant Canada. He prides himself on his English, especially the fact he speaks it with no detectable accent.

Salvador is twelve and, undeniably, extremely intelligent.

I didn't know Salvador was autistic when we first met. He seemed somewhat detached from what was going on around him, as his mother and I sat and discussed the family and the business she and her husband were engaged in, an enormously successful local cabaret and bar. Salvador's mother, Leticia, now had three children, having decided on a third only two years prior.

But the jewel in Leticia's estimable crown is undoubtedly Salvador. Before introducing me to this apparently distracted tween, she proudly told me of his academic achievements and her abiding suspicion that he was bound for inevitable greatness. She then told me that he was autistic and having let this sink in for a moment, introduced me to the strapping boy.

Salvador's eyes were bright and engaged and while it was clear he was reluctant to make eye contact with me, he did it. He did it because a concerted effort had been made to ensure that his autism wasn't going to hold him back. It had been assured that his social skills would be actively developed in order that he would be able to navigate the murky waters of social interactions without impediment.

There was an almost impish quality about him, but the composure and maturity of a boy so young was striking. When he opened his mouth and spoke to me in a virtually unaccented, flawless English, one might have knocked me over with a feather, so stunned was I by his verbal facility.

Early detection and diagnosis, a deeply engaged family unit and a commitment to Salvador reaching the fullness of his obviously vast potential, have all coalesced in a young, autistic man with a bright future. Salvador has no limitations, because he has been supported, encouraged and nurtured to embrace all he is and to live his dreams. Autism is only part of who he is. It doesn't define him.

Autistic people are as diverse as every other kind of person in the world. No two autistic people are exactly the same. Part of that is nature and part, nurture. There are so many determinants in play, it's difficult to point to either nature or nurture as the key to the success in the lives of people with autism. What I hope to illustrate with these three examples, though, is the role of support, encouragement and diagnosis in determining their quality of life. There is so much we can all do to make life better for people with this condition and I hope these examples have given you food for thought. I also hope that the diversity of the experience of the three, is instructional and provides hope for the future for those who live with autism reading this book. Let's look at some practical ways we can help people with autism thrive.

Helping an Autistic Loved One

As discussed above, autism is a spectrum which involves the manifestation of a wide range of symptoms in varying intensities and combinations. Knowing what the general symptoms are is a good starting point, but it's also important to know how they present in either you or a loved one. For the purposes of this section of the book, we'll assume you're a caregiver and talk about how you can support a loved one with the condition.

Observation is an important component of living with autism. Knowing your loved one's triggers in terms of symptomatic manifestations is important. What kinds of situations instigate meltdowns, zone outs, or aggression? What sends your autistic loved one off on a spree of repeating a phrase incessantly? Paying keen attention to what's happening immediately preceding a manifestation can help you head them off before it happens.

It's also important to observe what makes your autistic loved one happy. What are their pet interests? What causes them to withdraw into a quiet world of fascination? This could be the key to unlocking your loved one's unique gifts. In the case of Salvador, his facility with languages has been key, by involving him in a foreign exchange program. Your autistic love one has interests that can be developed into gifts that can translate into a future career.

In the case of an adult (depending upon the severity of symptoms), your loved one can find the kind of niches that Ricki and Bob found in their lives. Productive volunteering, community and support are all part of this. That means making sure the people around your loved one understand the symptoms in play, how they manifest and what causes them to manifest. This will make things easier for everyone.

Much of the advice on support in this book also applies to people with autism, regardless of age. Patience and understanding are the greatest gifts you can give people with autism. As I mentioned above, I was often challenged in that department with my friend, Bob. But because our interactions played out in a supportive environment, there were always others around to step in and get Bob moving and onto the business of the day, so I could get onto mine. Caregivers don't have this luxury, so it's important that you make sure you give yourself the opportunity to rest. Let someone else take the reins. A counsellor, or therapeutic professional, or art and music classes are good ways to achieve this effect. You need time for yourself and to remove yourself from the sometimes challenging world of autism. It can get pretty exhausting!

Self-care is important for those providing care and support to people with all the conditions discussed in this book, but because of autism's unique characteristics, it's even more important, if you're supporting a loved one struggling with it. Taking time for yourself and doing what you need to in order to recharge your batteries will keep you at your loved one's side, supporting and helping, for a long time to come. That means you need regular respite. Building this into your schedule is absolutely essential.

Respite (a moment of calm from the autism storm), can take as many forms as there are people. It may be a quiet couple of hours in the middle of your day while your charge it in a therapy session or class. It may be a visit to the gym, a long walk, or a trip to the spa. Respite could also mean finding a group of other caregivers to spend time with, share ideas and stories and also, discuss strategies for coping. Sometimes other people can help you find answers you might not on your own. It's always helpful to get a fresh perspective.

Whatever you do to re-charge yourself and find a little peace, make sure you're getting enough of it. Don't short yourself, because doing that isn't helping your loved one. You need to be well and at your best to go on this extended journey. The truth is that autism doesn't go away, just like with any of the other disorders described in this book. It's a lifelong challenge and that means you have to be equal to it. That means self-care and respite that honor the needs of your autistic loved one, by honoring your need for rest and rejuvenation.

Therapeutic Alternatives

The uniqueness of each person with autism makes finding the right therapy a challenge, but a combination of therapies which employ pharmaceuticals, clinical responses and alternative approaches will usually render symptom mitigation. Remember, autism doesn't "go away". It's there for life, so you're not looking for a cure. You're looking for a way to make life better for you, your loved one and the family you're both part of.

Applied Behavior Analysis

I've described this method of therapy in relation to other conditions, but it has a proven application in the support of autistic patients, as well. ABA is a collaborative therapy in which the patient's entire support network should be involved, in order to increase its effectiveness.

An educationally based therapy, ABA seeks to eliminate some of autism's more problematic symptoms and behaviors by linking reward to desired behaviors. Conversely, undesired behaviors are not punished, but not rewarded either. Once the patient is taught this in a consistent, systematic manner, improvements can be witnessed. This is true of children, youths and adults with autism.

In use since the 1960s, ABA techniques can be applied in every facet of life, from a structured classroom environment to the family breakfast table and social events. ABA can also be practiced in one on one therapeutic settings. It's proven successful in the development of social skills, promoting improved eye contact, listening without interrupting and learning not to blurt things out in church! The therapy is supported and recommended by many government agencies, including the US Surgeon General, as effective for all types of autism.

Greenspan Floortime Approach

This therapy model is entirely geared to young children and toddlers. Its aim is to bring forth the particular characteristics of individual children, encouraging them to move beyond diagnosis to a sense of self.

GFA encourages families to engage in baby-level play; to get down on the floor with them, in the midst of their toys and encounter them from their own perspective. GFA is ideal as a complement to other therapeutic approaches and can be employed in both clinical settings and the home.

This therapy allows the child to take the lead. Every child or toddler lives in a very unique, personal world of play and has favorite activities, toys and games. With parents and therapists entering into the child's imaginative world, insight into what baby enjoys is provided. Further, a sustained effort will allow increasing complexity of interaction and foster enhanced communications skills in the child.

GFA also supports early development in emotional thinking, self-regulation (control of emotions) and engagement with other people. This early intervention model is a unique way to bring autistic children out of their inner worlds and into the world of play, in which future social interactions are rooted. By allowing the patient to explore the world of play with others, socialization is set in motion. The child gains a sense of self through choosing the type of play to be pursued in therapy and parents gain a better understanding of how their autistic child sees the world.

Pivotal Response Treatment

An offshoot of ABA, PRT takes a similar approach to the GFA therapeutic method, in a play-based, child-led model. Supporting the development of language and communication, this approach is primarily for application to children older than those the GFA technique is designed for. PRT also helps children arrive at better regulation of autism symptoms that lead to disruptive behavior, through active socialization and aiding the development of two-way communication.

As its name suggests, PRT aims to impact those areas of a child's development which are pivotal to social interactions of all kinds.

These include social skills (including responses to social cues) and the ability to initiate social interaction. The model increases individual autonomy and agency by putting the child in the lead, while supporting the child's capacity for academic achievement through behavioral regulation.

While targeted to elementary school age children, PRT also has applications for older children and even young adults, due to the fostering of individual choice inherent to the therapy.

Verbal Behavior Therapy

VBT is another offshoot of ABA and seeks to improve communication skills, by helping patients learn to make linguistic connections between words, their purposes and their corresponding objects. Moving beyond the labelling of objects, VBT motivates patients to learn the reasoning behind language and to understand why words are used in making themselves understood as fully as possible.

The work of behavioral scientist B.F. Skinner forms the basis for this therapeutic model. Author of the book, *Verbal Behavior,* Skinner believed that dividing language in categories was the most efficient way to help autistic children make sense of it. In his model, the four categories employed are referred to as operants. Each has a different linguistic purpose, as follows:

- Mands are requests. A child might ask for a specific object.

- Tacts are indications that we want to share something, or to ask that someone look at what we're seeing. For example, pointing to a dog in the street.

- Intraverbals are responses to questions.

- An Echoic is an affirmative word in response to the same word being posed as a question.

Beginning with mands (requests), patients are taught that language elicits a desired response. Therapists repeat these requests to the patient, reinforcing the lesson by fulfilling the request, while repeating it. By feeding back language to the child, the effect is to build understanding of how language works, enhance interactive behaviors and teach the child the function of the different categories of language.

With mands being the most basic of the categories, the therapy builds on these, increasing the complexity through the various categories listed, with the effect that the child is ultimately able to apprehend the purpose of language and the connection of words to actions, objects and desired outcomes.

VBT is effective in reinforcing the positive results arising from the appropriate and consistent use of language. It's effective for both children and adults who struggle with verbal communication, especially those employing communication aids, like visual prompts, in order to communicate with others.

Early Intervention

I wonder how different Ricki's life might have been, had her autism been diagnosed when she was a child? How might she have developed differently if she'd had access to supportive therapy?

It's scientifically verifiable that early childhood intervention is an autistic child's best opportunity to development to the fullest potential possible. Every child won't respond in the same way to any of the models shown and results can vary as widely as the types and symptomatic make up of autism. All the same, early detection, diagnosis and therapy are strongly advised to achieve the best outcome possible. When seeking out therapies to help a child (or even an adult with autism), it's important that those ultimately chosen conform to certain recognized clinical and professional standards.

Regardless of the therapy chosen, the patient should be engaged in structured activities for twenty-five hours per week. This gives caregivers a welcome respite and provides the kind of professional clinical support people with autism need. This support should be provided by quality specialists in the field, with the help of support staff who are highly-trained in working with the symptoms of autism.

All therapies should be centered in addressing some of autism's most identifiable challenges, including impacts on language, the pursuit of play, fostering life skills and improving physical challenges like coordination. Socialization through sustained interaction should also be a primary goal.

Opportunities for peer and age group interaction is also important, as well as the involvement of parents. Parents should not be passive bystanders in any chosen therapy, but active participants who consult with therapeutic professionals in making treatment decisions. This facet of therapy indicates a general deference to parental desires about treatment delivery and places the family at the center of the model in play.

Finally, therapy for autistic people should always be pursued from a multidisciplinary standpoint. A team of professionals, according to the individual needs of the child, should be employed. Your family physician can assist you in assembling the right professionals to form a supportive team for your autistic loved one.

Alternative Therapies

There are many variations on the theme of alternative or complementary therapies out there for people with autism. Some are controversial, but where autism's concerned, a variety of treatments should be considered and none should be summarily dismissed. As counselled throughout this book, consulting a physician is always advised, prior to experimenting with supplements or other alternative therapies.

Prominent psychiatrist, Eric Hollander, counsels similarly. Dr. Hollander has seen people with autism make progress using complementary and alternative treatment. He tempers this assessment by saying there are possible side effects involved that should be taken into consideration. Also, trying too many things at once can muddy the waters in terms of benefit of the various therapies in play, to determine the effectiveness of any of them.

Casein-Gluten Elimination

Some parents and adults with autism claim to have seen results after eliminating casein (found in dairy products) and gluten (barley, wheat, rye) from the diet. While the benefits of this alternative treatment have not been clinically proven, trials are currently underway that may prove these claims.

While it's clear that the elimination of foods that contain these substances from the diet can do no direct harm, it's important that a nutrition and/or dietary specialist be consulted prior to implementation. The involvement of a clinical specialist in this area can ensure that those thinking about trying this strategy are taking into account the necessity for adequate nutrition to be delivered to the patient. Dairy and grains are nutritional building blocks and eliminating these foods from the diet can have health consequences, should replacement sources for the nutrients they provide not be sought.

The foods containing these substances are sources of necessary vitamins and also protein. Further, their elimination may have the potential to lead to deficiencies of zinc, Vitamin D and calcium (crucial for childhood bone development). Should the therapy be pursued, supplemental intake should be pursued to compensate for the elimination of the food sources in play.

Careful behavioral monitoring should be practiced while using this therapy and perhaps the re-introduction of one or the other of the food groups involved, if indicated by outcomes. Some report seeing improvement in behaviors like hyperactivity and disruptive behaviors by eliminating only foods containing casein. Others, with the elimination of foods containing gluten.

Starting with one or the other of the food groups implicated would be a measured approach to introducing this form of therapy. Concurrently, it's advisable to reduce or eliminate the intake of foods rich in processed sugar and fat, as these can exacerbate some of the symptoms of autism, as well.

Chelation

There has been a great deal of discussion about chelation therapy in the world of autism treatment, but I strongly advise that you not pursue this therapy.

The goal of this alternative therapy is to remove metals and other toxins from the body. Proponents suspect that these are introduced via pharmaceutical vaccines and may be responsible for the onset of autism. Mercury is pointed to as the chief culprit and those who promote this alternative therapy claim that its removal from the body via chelation "cures" autism.

As I said earlier in this chapter, there is no cure for autism. There are therapies which can ease symptoms and improve behaviors and quality of life, but there is no cure. Any therapy claiming to be a cure should be viewed with great suspicion.

Dr. James M. Laidler, once an enthusiastic supporter of chelation therapy, now refers to it as "quackery". He admits that his son's autism diagnosis sent him on a quest for a cure. He and his wife were driven to try a number of controversial or unproven therapies (including casein-gluten elimination, which is not yet scientifically proven to be effective in symptom reduction). The most controversial therapy they tried, though, was chelation, which they'd heard was a "miracle cure" for autism. Desperation makes people ignore their inner voices and that's what the Laidlers did in pursuit of the hope of a cure for their son's autism.

When a second child of the Laidlers was diagnosed with an ASD spectrum condition, they went into overdrive and by Dr. Laidler's own admission, tried as many alternative and complementary treatments as possible. In the process, they found themselves exhausted by it all, with two autistic children and no end (or progress) in sight.

Then, without Dr. Laidler's knowledge, his wife stopped a number of alternative therapies. There was no change in their children's behavior and this prompted them both to, eventually, drop the pursuit of alternative treatments for autism, opting instead for speech and behavioral therapy. As a result, both their children enjoyed steady improvement and the Laidler's were freed from the false claim that autism can be cured.

This is a cautionary tale for all those caring for loved ones with autism, or pursuing therapy for their own condition. It must always be remembered that autism is not curable; that it's a lifelong challenge. Any therapy which claims to be a silver bullet or miracle cure is be looked upon with a jaded eye.

The challenge of autism is its diversity. Every patient will respond differently and combinations of various therapies, trial and error and persistent investigation are what's needed. There's no easy way to do it. Observing the effects of various therapies is also necessary to determine what's working and what's not.

As I keep telling you, try a variety of therapies. Before you do, though, consult a medical professional. Don't gamble with your health, or that of your loved one. Take the time to do your homework and consult the right people. You'll get where you want to go with patience and persistence.

CHAPTER 7

HELPING CHILDREN WITH
SPECIAL NEEDS

Raising children with special needs is seen by many as a burden, but the truth is that it's more gift than burden. Children with special needs are unique, playful, funny and fascinated by the world around them, even though their relationship with it can be strained, at times. Their wonder can inform our own and make our lives richer by observing and participating in it.

This chapter will outline a number of ideas about how you can provide a nurturing, supportive environment for your special needs child. As always, trial and error will inform the choices you'll be making, as you become an expert in raising your special needs child.

Home schooling

Schooling special needs children at home is sometimes indicated, particularly in the case of autism (if symptoms are especially disruptive or severe). But it's not, by any means, appropriate for all special needs children. It can, in fact, be an isolating experience and a further strain on you and your support network. Pursuing education among other children is strongly advised, for its socializing effect and for the learning experiences available to special needs children in a group setting. Many school districts have services to support special needs children, so enquiring about these will make you aware of what's available in your area. Also, it must be understood that schooling at home represents a tremendous time investment on your part and frankly, you have plenty on your plate, already.

While homeschooling provides you with greater contact with your special needs child, that can come at a high price to both of you, as well as the rest of the family. It should only be pursued when absolutely necessary and with the guidance of an education assistant. Unless you're a professional educator, home schooling is not something you should pursue alone.

Turn down the pressure

While meaning well, parents sometimes put too much pressure on their children to succeed, without knowing they're doing it. This can be true of parents with special needs children, too. The problem is that this pressure can impede progress and success and breed frustration for both parents and children. Patience, as stated throughout this book, is what's required, even if it means your child's development takes longer than you might like. The involvement of educational professionals in either your home schooling plan, or in the public education system is strongly advised. These professionals can guide your strategies, working with your child and passing on valuable information on to you, as they have a unique perspective. Also highly useful are clinical professionals. They are trained to work with special needs children and their input can help prevent the parental tendency to ask too much of their children.

By the same token, parents of special needs children ask a great deal of themselves. This should be tempered by calling on the crucially important support of professionals and the supportive network of friends, family and others who can help.

Encourage

Encourage your child to pursue activities that produce happiness. Happiness is a balm for special needs children, so it's important that they do those things that optimizes it. When your child achieves a goal, completes a task, or does things without your help, praise is the most supportive help you can give. Recognizing even the smallest achievement (even just getting into bed without your prompting) is a big part of building the confidence and self-esteem of special needs children. Apply it lavishly, regularly and as a way of life.

Independence

All parents want to do things for their children, but unless children (especially special needs children) learn to do things on their own, they won't develop to their full potential. As mentioned previously, resist making all decisions for your child. Children need to develop independence by doing things themselves. From an early age, it's important to instill in them the understanding that they're their own best friend and that they're capable of doing many things on their own. The sense of ownership this provides all children is very important for special needs children, as well. This might be a tough thing to do as a parent, but it is something that will help your child develop the independence necessary to develop necessary life skills.

Don't worry

Moms and dads worry. It goes with the territory. It doesn't have to be a way of life, though and frankly, shouldn't be. It changes nothing, except your enjoyment of life and your special needs child. Give it up as a lifestyle, if you're indulging in it that intensely. Remember that your frame of mind has an impact on your child's quality of life. Children sense things and special needs children can be particularly sensitive to the moods and attitudes of people around them.

Be Selective About Media

There is a lot of information out there these days. The world is full of media on a 24/7, 365 cycle and a lot of it is completely unsuitable for children. For this reason, it's important that you be aware of what your child is being exposed to. This is even more important in the case of special needs children. It's vital that you curate the media your child is exposed to and discourage anything that might have a negative, or even harmful impact. Certain content, especially if it's violent, frightening, or otherwise negative, can have a lasting impact on children. Make sure that what your child is exposed to is positive, educational and useful.

Key Take Aways

Informing yourself about the condition you or your loved one is suffering from is one of the key tools in your toolbox. With knowledge, you can approach the condition systematically and intelligently. Be sure to use reliable resources in your studies, as misinformation is dangerous. It can mislead you as to the appropriateness of therapies and accompanying medications and may impede progress for you or your loved. Life with any of these conditions is difficult enough, without adding incorrect information to your woes. Read as much about the condition as you can. Create a Google alert to get the latest information on research and emerging therapies, so you're up to date and don't miss out on new developments.

Seek out allies and build a network of support around you. Family, friends, neighbors, co-workers and clinical professionals should all be part of your network. Everyone you know has a part to play. Part of creating a support network is your willingness to share what you know about the condition with the people in it. This will strengthen your network and make its connections stronger and more effective.

Don't suffer in silence. Reach out and enlist the support you need. You're only one person. While it can be humbling to reach out and ask for help, you need to take this step to keep your sanity and wellbeing intact. Open up to those around you and share your struggles. If people don't know about what you face in your day to day life with the condition, or living with someone who has it, how can they hope to help and support you?

There will always be those around us who don't get it. They either don't believe that the condition exists, or they believe it's a made up product of modernity – just another thing for people to bitch about. These are not the sort of friends and allies you need. Keep your distance. People with attitudes like these are the problem, not the solution. They're never going to understand, so don't waste your time trying to get through to them. Concentrate on cultivating the positive relationships around you.

Patience is not only a virtue. Patience has to be the foundation of your relationship with a loved who has any of the conditions mentioned in this book. Asperger's, ADHD and autism are challenging conditions that can fray the nerves of the people around patients who have them. Patience will be your biggest gift to a loved one with one of these conditions. Not everyone is able to model it in the presence of these conditions, but your loved one needs you to.

But you're not a saint. You're going to lose it every now and again. You're not made of iron, either. There will be times when you'll feel exhausted. This is where your support group is so important. As a caregiver, you need respite. You can't possibly be expected to remain in service 24 hours a day. There are times you'll need to step away to do what you need to, but also to rest and rejuvenate yourself. Burning out is not an option. So self-care is something you need to do. It's not just for you. It's for your loved one, also. If you're not there, because you're sick or burned out, life will be much more difficult.

Diet plays a very important role when it comes to treating children with Asperger's, ADHD or autism. Removing processed and junk foods from your loved one's diet is key to managing symptoms, as these can exacerbate the situation. A fresh, balanced diet, incorporating the fundamental food groups (vegetables, fruit, dairy, grain, proteins) should feature all the nutrients we've discussed earlier in this book. Iron, zinc and magnesium are extremely important to the health and functioning of the brain, so be sure to incorporate as many sources of these into the family diet as you're able. Omega 3 fatty acids are another dietary support that should be present in combatting any of these conditions. If you're going to try an elimination diet, like dairy or grain elimination (or both, concurrently), check with your family doctor first and make you're your loved one is receiving sufficient nutrition.

Supplements can also play an important role in symptom management, as described earlier. It's very important, though, that your physician be consulted to ensure that you're choosing the right ones and that your choices are not going to interact negatively with other medications in play. Be sure that these are easily digestible and from natural sources. Additives in supplements are something to be considered, so be sure to read the label.

Exercise is a cornerstone of good health and a life practice everyone should engage in. This is especially true for people who live with Asperger's, ADHD, or autism. Physical activity releases the hormone, serotonin. This is another important, naturally-occurring chemical in the body which promotes brain health and a sense of wellbeing. Serotonin also acts to suppress cortisol, the chemical released in the body when we're depressed or stressed.

Engaging in a sport or outdoor activity can be liberating for people who suffer from these conditions and distract them from some of their symptoms. The release of physical exercise is good for everyone, but serves a functional purpose when added to other therapies to address these conditions. If you choose a sport, there is the added benefit of group activity, involving cooperation with other people. For any of the three conditions discussed, this can promote enhanced social skills and answer some of the self-isolating tendencies people with them face. Being with other people is an important therapeutic factor for those with any of these conditions.

Hobbies are a wonderful way for people with Asperger's, ADHD and autism to find relief from their symptoms. By channeling some of the love of detail these conditions tend to feature into a hobby that indulges them, the patient can also find great satisfaction. Pursuing a hobby that fits the clinical reality of these conditions (model-building, for example) frames them in a more positive light. These conditions become positives and not negatives, because the symptoms reveal themselves as having a useful application. They're good for something!

Whether you have one of these conditions, or a loved one does, finding a hobby that most aptly reflects the symptomatic gifts involved can be liberating and validating. Some autistic people, for example, are known to have special gifts in the realm of music and the arts. Finding our passion is part of life's journey and one of its most uplifting aspects. Finding your personal passion, or that of your loved one, can completely change the way the world looks. It can become a place of joy, no longer threatening or confusing.

People who suffer from Asperger's, ADHD and autism need understanding, patience and above all, love. A sense of belonging and the knowledge that they're not alone are positives in the life of people living with the challenges presented by these conditions. That includes you, if you're the one with the condition. If you're living with any of these conditions through a loved one, though, the difference you can make in that person's overall quality of life is immeasurable. Check in with yourself regularly to assess how things are going. Be honest, at times when you're worn out by it all. Most of all, consider the experience you're in the midst of to be one which builds your character and sense of self. Self-awareness and honesty about your weaknesses are deeply important. If you're caring for a loved one, know that the rewards of the experience are far greater, ultimately, than the challenges. You're on a unique, collaborative journey. Embrace it, learn from it and grow.

The ride can be wild, challenging and illuminating, all at the same time. What matters most is that you or your loved one come to an understanding of the condition you're working with and how best to manage its symptoms. Diligent application of therapeutic remedies will help, but it's most important that your approach be positive, at all times. Building yourself up is part of it. Learning to process what can be negative symptoms into learning and even professional success (because there are positives that can lead to work in analytical fields in the cases of all conditions covered here) is one of the outgrowths of living with these conditions. Look for those opportunities actively, each day.

CONCLUSION

Thank you again for purchasing this book!

I hope its' contents were able to help you understand autism, Asperger's syndrome, and ADHD a little better.

My main goal in writing this book was to educate people about the challenges of these conditions and how understanding them can make life not only easier, but more successful for those living with them. I hope I was able to provide you with the kind of information that will enable you to do that and to thrive, as you live with these sometimes difficult conditions.

The next step is for you to apply these strategies. Remember you're on a journey that can be a struggle at times, even stressful. But it can also be one of the most rewarding and fulfilling experiences you've ever had. Remember to continue to learn and grow as you move along the path and to cherish the struggle as a gift, above all.

Finally, if you enjoyed this book, then I'd like to ask a favor. Would you be kind enough to leave a review for this book on Amazon? I'd very much appreciate it!

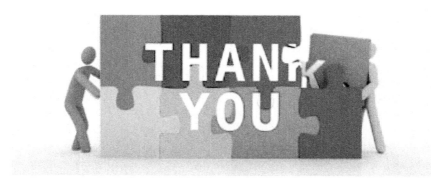

BONUS:

Enjoy this bonus video

https://www.youtube.com/watch?v=YeWks6cgJ-k

CPSIA information can be obtained
at www.ICGtesting.com
Printed in the USA
LVOW04s0045220416
484724LV00028B/503/P

9 781515 030508